# THE BOOK ON
# SITUATIONAL
# AWARENESS

Live with More Peace and Confidence

# THE BOOK ON
# SITUATIONAL
# AWARENESS

## Actionable Tips and Exercises
## to Protect Your Personal Safety

# MATT PATRICK KELLY

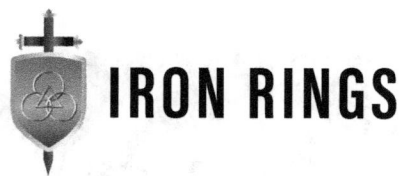

# IRON RINGS

ISBN: 979-8-218-14065-6 (Print)
ISBN: 979-8-218-14066-3 (E-Book)

Cover Design: Style-Matters.com
Cover Imagery: Shutterstock/your

*To the two most important women in my life—my amazing wife, Angie, and my daughter, Cynia—your beauty, intelligence, creativity and examples of being amazing humans have taught me more than I could ever explain. The love, blessings, and joy you both have gifted me in this life can only be summed up as, "my cup runneth over." And to my son, Justin, whose zest for life, contagious smile, humor, and positive outlook on life are true blessings to mine.*

# CONTENTS

# TOP TIER 133

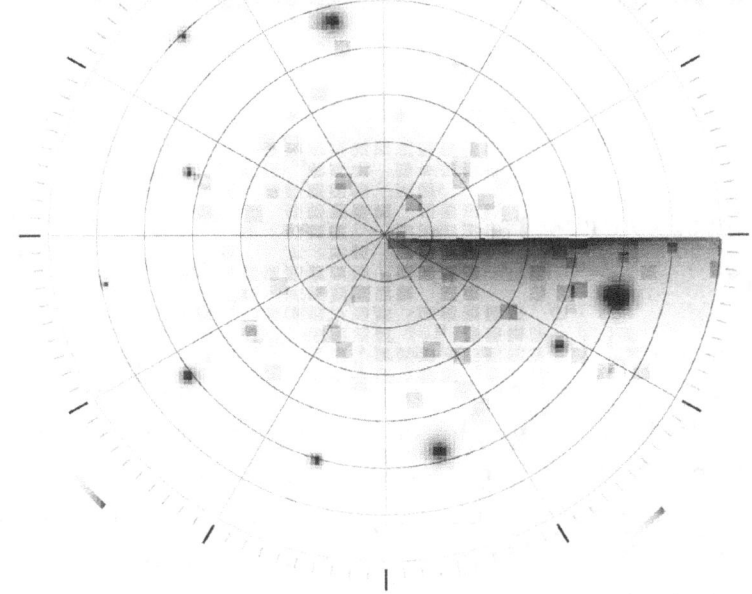

# ACKNOWLEDGMENTS

Special thanks to Clint Smith, Tim Kennedy, Jacko Willink, Mike Kurcina from Spotter-Up, Andy Curtiss, Mickey Schuch with Carry Trainer, Zevon Durham (a.k.a. "Instructor Zee"), Mike Glover with Fieldcraft Survival, and Karl Erickson with Tactical Rifleman. The great thing about writing a book is that you get to give shout-outs to some of your heroes. The men mentioned above are top-tier in my list of heroes.

Thank you for being caring and empathetic teachers for people from all walks of life. By your words and actions you've inspired and driven me to become a better person, and I know you've positively impacted countless others. As Zee would say, "Keep choppin' wood."

My must-have shout-outs: I have to absolutely applaud and thank, a million times over, my project manager, Anna Krusinski, for teaming up with me on this work! Thank you, Anna, for editing this work, and for taking my "brain vomit" and making this passion project of mine flow with much more ease, tone, and clearer and more concise messaging. I must also thank you for leading me through the entire process as a "rookie" author, from first draft all the way through print and publishing! Thank you also for teaming me up with Bob Murray at StyleMatters, who spearheads success for authors from all walks of life and who graciously hooked me up with Jerry Dorris, the graphic designer for this book's cover design, book layout, and overall feel for this work. You all are amazing humans; you are all subject-matter experts in your fields. It must be said that one of the most enjoyable parts of getting this project completed was having the stars align so I had the honor and privilege to work with you all. You all have damn near broken my gratitude meter!

Super bonus special thanks to my brothers-in-arms who always tell me the truth (even if it will hurt) and do me favors not out of score-keeping but out of true caring and love. They navigate this modern complexity with me, and we all have each other's best interests at heart. They have my six whenever needed, regardless of time, place, or inconvenience. Rob Leahy, Dr. John A. King, Bill Aycock, Bryan Deemer, and last but never least, Billy D., one William Dolentz. This collection of great men with knowledge ranging from personal safety, self-protection, literature, history, religion, SWAT operations, law enforcement, and hunting have all vetted this content. They are fathers, brothers, sons, and husbands. They, like myself, will stop at nothing to protect, train, and empower each and every aspect of life that is precious to them. We humbly count ourselves among the dying class of real men in this modern era. It is with our collective love and best wishes that you find this work helpful, insightful, challenging, exhilarating, and yet fun to learn. Please enjoy!

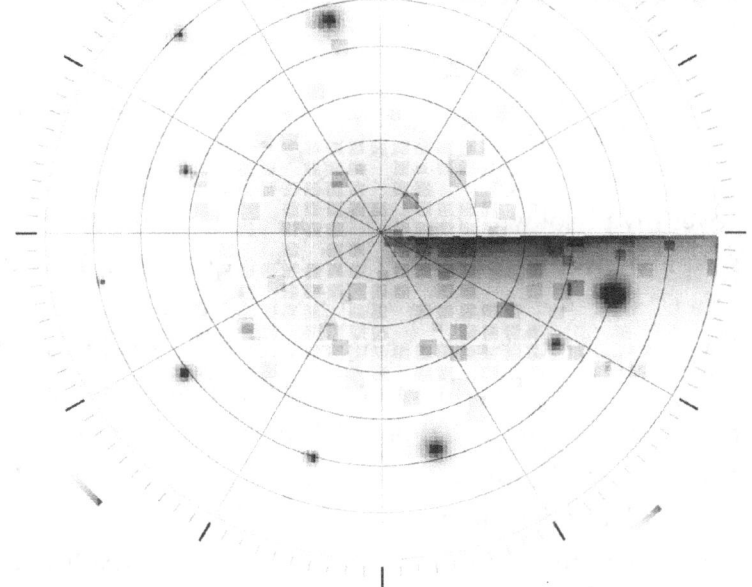

# INTRODUCTION

S ituational awareness is knowing where you are and what is going on around you, allowing individuals and organizations to be more alert and informed and to make better and safer decisions. Here are a few examples from my own life: I was a twenty-three-year-old Dallas rookie police officer working solo in a squad car while making a traffic stop in one of the worst, crime-riddled beats (Beat 243) in the city. The vehicle I pulled over had out-of-date registration, with one lone male occupant as the driver. As I slowly approached the vehicle, I noticed the man was intently focused on the small driver's-side rearview mirror and he was watching my approach, *timing* my approach. As I got close to the rear of the car, to approach the driver's-side window, I saw his body weight shift, ever so slightly. It was a slight sway, left to right, and I saw his right shoulder was perched a few inches higher than what might seem normal or relaxed. Something didn't feel right, and I knew this could go very bad. Knowing he was watching me, I let him see me cover my pistol with my dominant hand, unsnapping the retention straps so my gun could be unholstered quickly, if needed. With my other hand, I grabbed my handheld radio and called for backup as I moved behind the rear of his car, to the right-side passenger door of my squad car. Backup came, a two-man unit, and we performed a felony stop. As it turned out, this man had violated his parole, had a warrant out for his arrest, and was in possession of a .357 revolver that he had been moving around and trying to get into position when I had first approached. Situational awareness has saved my life on countless occasions. As another example, I was working with a female HR professional who shared with me after one of my active-shooter classes that she had been alone on an elevator one time, and as the doors started to close, a man (whom she hadn't seen before, when she got on the elevator) jabbed his hand into the closing door of the elevator at the last second and entered the elevator with her. She immediately felt this man was up to no good, and she darted off the elevator and hurried toward a group of people at the front desk in the lobby. I applauded her for her situational awareness and trusting her instincts and intuition, and I told her that I truly believe she had saved herself from an unwanted situation.

We all have situational awareness, so no one reading this work is starting from zero. Some readers, whether by occupation, trade, or personal experience, will have more situational awareness than others. And some readers, being untouched by violence and the multitude of distractions our modern era presents, will have less awareness while navigating through their daily lives. No matter where you are, no matter how much awareness you have or don't have, know that more is always better in this case.

Our skills and abilities are perishable. So, to stay relevant and up to speed, it is wise to have some form of scheduled time or routine in place to practice and keep yourself sharp—and safe. If you've had some experience with building situational awareness in the past but you've let those skills dull over time with lack of practice, this will probably be a quick journey to get you back to where you want to be, back to your "level set." And if you're new to this, keep in mind that regular practice will be your key to success as you learn how to execute these skills.

Staying sharp and practiced is crucial to protecting your personal safety and the safety of those you love. Make time to make practice happen! Lack of time is an excuse I often hear when it comes to putting forth meaningful effort to accomplish one's goals, hone their skills, and increase their abilities. But the truth is, this is simply a personal choice: to do or not do. Excuses don't matter; they're irrelevant. Focusing on one concept or group of exercises each week should allow plenty of wiggle room for you to get in some value-added skill-building without taking over your life. We all have the same twenty-four hours in a day. What separates the successful from the unsuccessful is what they do within that same amount of time we all share.

This book is structured so you can read a chapter each week and then work on the drill(s), exercises, and/or scenarios by practicing them daily throughout the week. At the end of each chapter is a card that could be photographed on a smartphone to be used as a quick reference of the material. So, a chapter could be read and the card associated with that chapter could be kept on your phone as a reminder of that week's situational exercise. If you follow this weekly format, this book will provide a year's worth of practice. The chapters can be done in order, or you can pick and choose based on the titles or in a random order at the start of each week. You could also read the book from cover to cover and then decide which chapter(s) you want to focus on.

Rome wasn't built in a day, and it will take time to build up the brain muscle (neural pathways) that will enable each exercise to become a natural way of thinking and acting in your daily life. Preparation isn't based in fear of what could go wrong. Preparation is, by definition, *the action or process of making ready or being made ready for use or consideration.* Preparation, as in, being prepared or being a "prepper," seems to have a lot of negative associations these days. Preppers are often thought of as conspiracy theorists, wack-jobs, weirdos, and paranoid folks who live in fear. To me, this couldn't be further from the truth. Preparation is a natural course of life that we all do. Have you ever "prepared" for a test or exam so you would do well, rather than just leaving it to chance? Being prepared is smart and meaningful. Having the wherewithal and the tools (especially mental ones) ready for use or consideration is being smart. It is the intent of this book to provide actionable exercises to help you develop or enhance skills that can be built upon to allow you to live with more peace and confidence as you navigate your daily life.

It is my hope that you never have to employee these techniques during a natural or man-made situation or disaster. However, knowing these techniques—and training in their execution on a daily basis—will better prepare you should a negative unpredictable outcome ever arise. This will put you miles ahead of where you would be if you had never given it prior consideration, thought, practice, or execution, because trying to think and act clearly while the "lead is flying" means you're already behind the proverbial eight ball.

Each chapter is written with public settings in mind (unless there is a specific reference), *but* it can't be overlooked or understated that each of these *should* be given equal consideration—in their preparation and practice—in the workplace, at home, on vacation, while traveling, during overnight hotel stays, etc. So, within the framework of practicing one chapter each week, if you multiply that by three (for public, work, and personal settings), then this book has at least 156 points for you to drive home in just one short year. To some this might sound like homework, but protecting your life— and the lives you can positively affect by learning to live situationally aware—should be the most important "work" you do to continue living and enjoying all the positive things you can experience.

It is with every best wish for a positive outcome that I have been driven to create this work for those with no experience, those with some experience, and even for the high-speed, low-drag badasses out there who just want to keep their edges razor-sharp.

All my best,

MATT PATRICK KELLY

FOUNDER OF THE KNIGHT'S PATH (HTTPS://WWW.THEKNIGHTSPATH.COM)

# BASIC

...................................................................................................

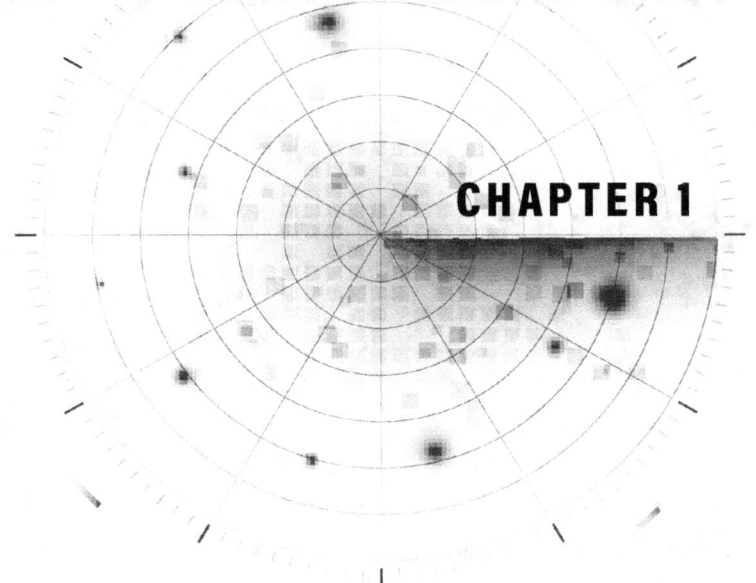

# CHAPTER 1

# EXITS

**Two questions:**

1. Can an exit save your life? This week's exercise can (and should) be quite the task. Think of every place you inhabit throughout the week. If there are ten places this week, then you will have some work to do.
2. When is the next active shooter event going to happen? No one knows! They are unpredictable and can happen in what we consider random places (but, oftentimes, they're *not* random to the planner or active killer of these evil deeds). I think you get the point...do your homework!

## Exercise:

In all buildings (public and private), stores, or facilities you find yourself in (or about to go into), know the number of exits and where they are located. Once the exits have been determined, rank them as contingencies: A, B, C, or 1, 2, 3. For example: Plan A, I will go to this exit because it is the closest to me with the least amount of people to move around to get out of this structure. Plan B, if Plan A is not an option (because there are bad guys there, or because a doorway is jammed with people), I will exit the structure here. Plan C, if Plans A and B aren't viable, then I will exit this third way to safely escape this structure. Don't forget about fire exits! (You know, the ones with signage that says "Don't exit or the alarm will sound.")

## Purpose:

The reason you want at least three contingencies is because pre-thought places a mental "bullet" in your chamber, ready to fire (act out) when/if the SHTF (shit hits the fan). The purpose of this is for you to have already baked in a mental go-to upon which you can more immediately react, instead of being surprised by the thing(s), person, or people causing the shit to hit the fan.

Without pre-thought (and visualization, which will be covered later), you'd be trying to think clearly and react appropriately in a high-stress environment in real-time while the lead is flying, and your chance for success under these circumstances drops significantly. You'll be at a disadvantage, a slave to lag time and the action-beats-reaction principle. You will be behind the proverbial eight ball, which means panic can easily ensue and your brain will potentially draw from its short-term memory the last thing it remembers, which is that the exit is the entrance. This makes sense to your brain because the entrance is the place by which you got in, so that is where you would also need to get out. Most people will likely be in this group (if they aren't frozen in their tracks), and those who snap to attention after initially freezing will be looking for leadership and guidance and could easily follow other folks who are trying to react appropriately but are all moving in a similar direction. This scenario would cause a flooding school of fish, or a herd mentality, of people rushing to one place, which won't be the best option if an active shooter is in a room and is trying to kill as many people as they can and stack their head count.

If I'm a bad guy and I think like a bad guy (more on this later, too), and my sole aim is to kill as many innocents as possible, then I'm going to be focused on the greatest mass and concentration of people. The eyes are attracted to and will key in on movement—and this goes for good people and bad guys. Having A, B, and C contingencies to escape a building with pre-thought could mean the difference between being a lone Atlantic bluefin tuna that breaks away from the school to be ignored by the predator versus becoming a target that's easy to hit, like shooting fish in a barrel.

## Things to Consider:

Wouldn't it be good to know prior to entry where your exits are, versus being dependent upon a posted evacuation map that is *hopefully* accurate, clearly labeled, and conveniently posted to give you this information? Perhaps a drive around the parking lot or a walk around the building or structure would be a wise course of action to confirm your contingencies upon entry.

## Bonus:

If there is a kitchen, it more than likely has an exit (or exits). For example, food courts in malls have hidden trash and delivery hallways to bring things to and from. These are not often

considered when contemplating exits, so ponder this well during
your weekly exercise.

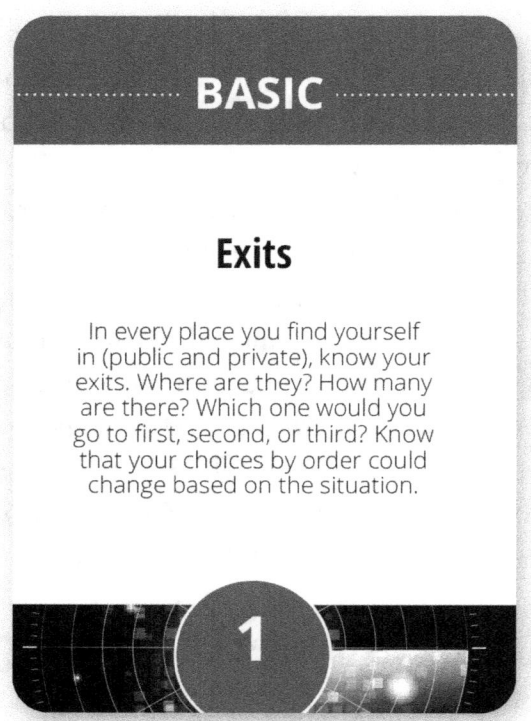

**BASIC**

**Exits**

In every place you find yourself
in (public and private), know your
exits. Where are they? How many
are there? Which one would you
go to first, second, or third? Know
that your choices by order could
change based on the situation.

1

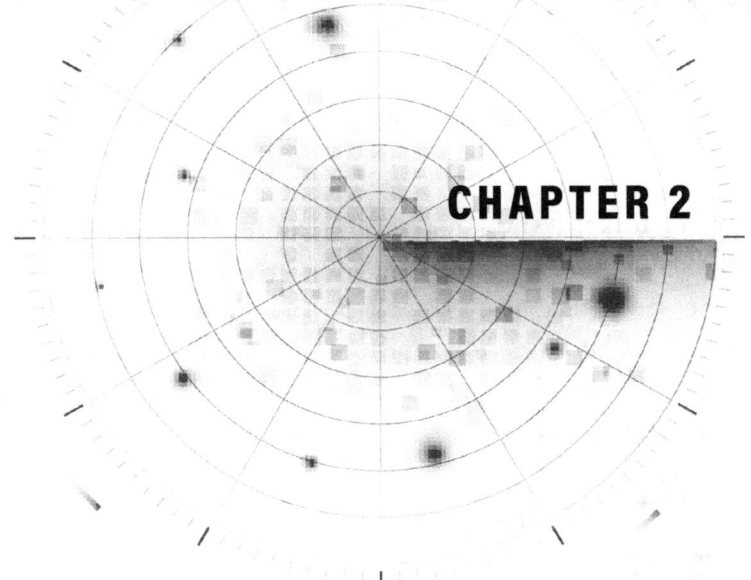

# CHAPTER 2

# CREATURE OF HABIT (DON'T BE ONE)

**T**his chapter is all about alternate routes. This is a teaser and "pre-work" to Chapter 25: Oswald Is Coming, but it's a great launching point.

## ⚙ Exercise:

Discover and *practice* three to five alternate routes to and from work and public outings. Make sure to use different routes there and back; don't take an alternate route to your destination and then take the same alternate route back, just because it's not the norm. If you do, you're becoming a creature of habit. Here's an uncomfortable pretend-stalker thought: "Oh, the lady I'm stalking took a different route to work and the same one home...good to know; if she takes a different route to work, she'll likely take the same one home. I know just where to set up my camera for some sweet facial shots I'll use privately in my bathroom later." I think you get it, folks! (And for the guys reading this...just 'cause that little stalker story was gal-focused doesn't mean you're immune. Males who see you as the obstacle to their undying female obsession— whether because you're the boyfriend, husband, or protective brother—could track and target your creature habits, as well. You're not exempt, so *do the drill*!)

## ✚ Bonus:

Look at a map first and memorize the routes. Phones can go down and computers can go down, so you need to commit the routes to memory. Buy a paper map. (I know, they are rare!) Also, once you've got three or more routes, decide which one you would prefer to walk if you had to.

### Extra Bonus:

Do you have a "get home" bag? (A "get home" bag is a bag with the tools and supplies to get you home safely, should your car break down (as just one example). It would typically include food, water, a battery charger for your phone, flashlight, etc.) What would you fill it with? What should you fill it with?

## BASIC

# Creature of Habit (Don't Be One)

Do you take the same path to and from work each day? Mix it up by finding and practicing three to five alternate routes to and from places during the week. Stalkers, weirdos, and criminals want you to be predictable!

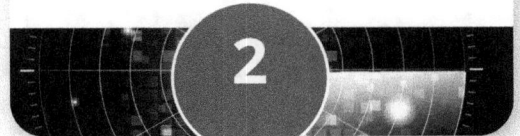

**2**

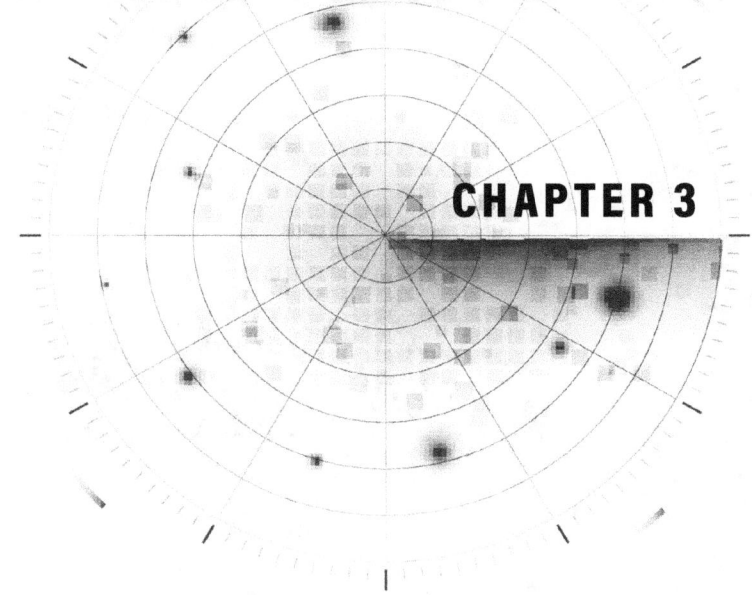

# CHAPTER 3

# ODD MAN OUT

Pick out the oddball or something that doesn't "fit." It can be as small as a person with a face tattoo or a scarf, or someone with super expensive pumps. The point is to notice something that stands out when compared to the regulars in this place and space. We'll build upon this in a later chapter.

### Exercise:

As you go through your week of daily activities, pick out someone or something that is unusual, seems out of place, or is simply different. This could be as obvious as someone who is dressed in wedding attire while shopping at a convenience store, or it could be something more challenging and harder to notice, like someone with a pierced earlobe without an earring in it.

## BASIC

### Odd Man Out

Look for something unusual about someone in a crowd. This is training you for discernment. It can be anything from someone who's wearing five-inch stilettoes or a jacket in summer to fine details such as someone with a pierced hole in a nose or eyebrow but no ring in that space.

**3**

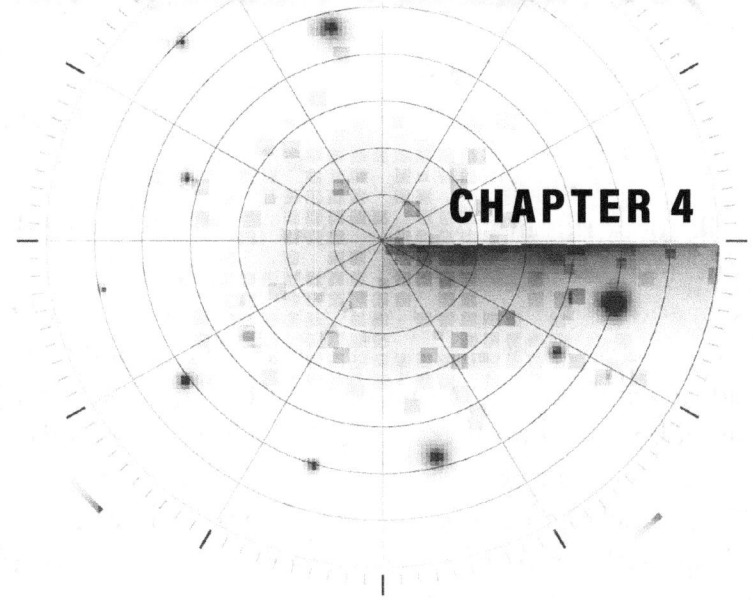

# CHAPTER 4

# TO THE CAR

admit, sometimes I'm driving down the interstate, with my eyes open and looking forward, operating a motor vehicle at seventy miles per hour, looking completely aware and in control with the act of driving that I'm performing, when I look up at some point and realize, *Crap! I just passed my exit!* Obviously, I then have to take the next exit, adjusting my course to get back on track for the destination I originally had planned. Now, tell me if this hasn't happened to you on one or more occasions. In the example above, I was heading home and it was a lock, a no-brainer; I'd done it hundreds of times, easy peasy, no *problemo*, right?! Wrong! You see, I was paying bills in my head, culling through honey-dos, or engaging in a multitude of other mental distractions that can get in the way of living in the present moment, being completely situationally aware, and giving my full attention to the action I was performing at the time, which was twofold: 1) Drive well, while being aware. 2) Get home safely and unscathed, i.e., arrive alive. I'll talk about this in more detail in Chapter 36: Shock the Monkey, but for now, just know that I wasn't paying full attention. It is so easy for us to get distracted in our daily lives, with all that's going on, with all the bombardments we receive second by second from advertisements, cell phone notifications, signage, radio, podcasts, audiobooks, to-do lists, paying bills in our head, or dealing with unruly kiddos who are fighting in the back seat while you're trying to get safely home. The truth is, it happens all the time to all of us. Snap to it! Get your head in the game for this week's exercise.

## Exercise:

At least once each day of the week, assume someone is following you! Use Chapter 42: Walk the Walk, Chapter 43: Vision Quest, and any others in this book which you deem fit, to determine if someone is on your 6 o'clock (following you). Can they run up to you and play Tag, You're It (from Chapter 41) as you get your vehicle's door open? Not to worry so much if it's a mother of five trying to corral her kiddos into the minivan parked next to you. But if you notice a sketchy character, then *abort, abort, abort!* You don't have to go to your car; you can look around as if you forgot where it was parked. You can go to the cart corral, throw away your receipt, and bide some time to see what they do. Surround yourself with a bubble of space before you enter your vehicle. A douchebag in a vehicle parked next to yours should be an ultra-warning sign, but there's nothing wrong with getting in from the passenger's side door or the back door, even if you then have to shimmy up to the driver's seat to make your vehicular exit. Also, there's nothing wrong with accidentally hitting your car alarm—*oops!*—to draw attention to your area before your clumsy self safely gets in, locks the door, and makes it home.

Obviously, I *don't* want anyone to actually follow you! I threw some of those details in because it could happen, and I wanted to give you some things to consider prior to performing this exercise. In a perfect world (but it isn't), this exercise would be performed with low stress, and you would be able to ensure you have a good bubble of space around you and you are situationally aware of your surroundings as you get to your car, put away your groceries, and perhaps get that kiddo securely placed in their car seat. Definitely couple this with Chapter 52: Establish Ownership. In fact, please skip ahead and get familiar with that exercise ASAP because it is, in my opinion, one of the most important ones in this book.

## Things to Consider:

Have your keys already in your hand so you can quickly get into your car and then immediately lock your doors. Fumbling around in a pocket or digging around in your purse can eat up precious bits of time that could be better served getting you into the protected environment of your ride—and it's more difficult to assault a car than a person.

## BASIC

### To the Car

If you were in a store and were told someone was following you, how aware would you be as you went back to your car? As you go to your car, subtly raise your awareness as if someone were following you. If this were true, what would you do?

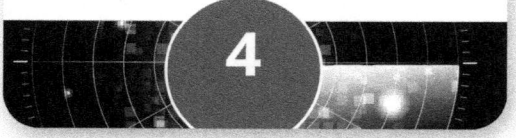

4

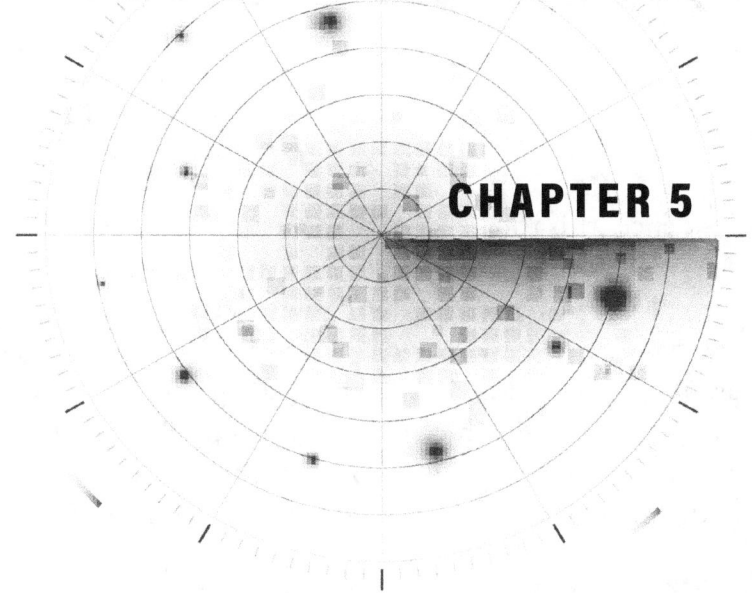

# CHAPTER 5

# TO THE CASA

**T**his is a great combo with Chapter 4: To the Car. So, you made it to the car safe and sound, and now you're heading home...

## Exercise:

Assume someone is following you from a public setting as you're heading home. You're ten miles from home, and with some rear-facing mirror awareness, you notice that a white panel van with no windows, three cars back, changes lanes when you do and exits when you exit. If you think someone *is* following you, then *don't go home*! This would only show them where you live. If this truly were the case, you'd instead want to pass your house, make some turns, and determine if they are still following you. If they are, head to a police station or fire station while calling 911. I don't recommend going to a friend or loved one's place of residence; this then becomes a location of interest and an area for the stalker to stake out.

As with To the Car, I don't want this to be the case. Preferably, this would be a low-stress drill where you will become more acutely aware of what is around you and trailing you as you head to places. In a perfect world (which it's not), this will allow you to confirm that no bad characters are following you. This is also a perfect piggyback with Chapter 14: Blue Four-Door Sedan with Texas Plates.

## Things to Consider:

Just like in To the Car, have your keys in your hand so that you can quickly get in your home and lock the door. Scanning your environment prior to approaching the threshold is also a wise move. Having bushes and shrubbery around your home's entrance might look visually appealing, but it could also present great places for bad people to hide. Think about these things when you're dolling up that curb appeal for your humble abode. Also, *ditch* the key hidden under a fake rock or welcome mat or perched on a ledge that seems hard to reach, etc. It wouldn't take long for a stalker to watch your house and see your neighbor unwittingly reveal where the "hidden" spot is when you've called them to walk your dog because you had to stay late at the office.

And finally, for all you shooters out there: When you're leaving the gun range, you could be followed. They *know* you have weapons, and depending on your state (such as New Jersey, which has turd gun laws), you might have to lock your gun in a case and separate the ammo from the gun. So, a bad person with ill intent might follow you, case you, and find out where you live for a later burglary—if they don't hit you when you pull in the driveway. No-brainer here, but bad guys don't give a *hoot* about gun laws.

And now, a personal share on grocery shopping and making multiple trips to and from your dwelling. When I was a Dallas police officer, I responded to a case where two young college students had been making multiple trips carrying groceries to and from the car to their first-floor apartment. The rapist timed the women's last trip from the car to the apartment (which was easy to do with a trunk close and an alarm chirp), then, as the last young woman turned to shut the door, she was pushed inside. He then locked the door and began what would end up being four or five hours of horror for these two young women. After gagging and restraining the women with common household items (such as electrical extension cords, T-shirts, and dish towels), this scourge to human existence raped and terrorized these two innocent women multiple times over the course of the next several hours. This is hard for me to write, but if there is any silver lining to point out in this criminal act, it is this: he didn't murder them. He performed his evil acts and left them bound and gagged, then he unlocked the front door, closed it behind him, and left. One of the brave young women escaped her bonds, unbound her roommate, and then called the police. I was one of the first officers to respond. We gathered a suspect description, communicated this over the airwaves, and soon had several officers searching the area. Detectives and crime scene technicians soon responded. These two young women were survivors, and they were extremely brave while being able to gather their wits after what they had experienced to answer my questions and give me the information I was asking for. I could see and feel the palpable effects of their traumatic experience, especially as the minutes and hours went by. Twenty-eight years later, I can still see their faces. They were beautiful, young, innocent women. I can hear their broken voices, and it makes me sad, breaks my heart, and infuriates me—all at once, and once again. This case has left its mark on my soul. I have shared this story numerous times to women young and old.

The main takeaways are to be aware and have a plan. Making multiple trips from a vehicle into a house or an apartment is a point of vulnerability. This criminal seized upon this vulnerability. I want to be clear: I'm not finding fault with these two women; they absolutely didn't deserve what happened to them. Thousands of women perform these acts every day and suffer no ill effects. However, there are some principles, tactics, and strategies to be learned from this. There is no right or wrong answer, and there is no guarantee that if these lessons had been used the negative outcome wouldn't have happened anyway. Keeping this in mind, here are some tips to help prevent this type of scenario:

- Lock the door between trips to and from the house.
- Have one person (if there are two or more) as a lookout, with cell phone in hand, and with 911 dialed and ready to hit send.
- Minimize your trips. If it can be done in one trip, then this means less "exposure." *But* this also will likely mean that all the things you're carrying could become a distraction (you're focusing on the eggs and bread not being crushed rather than keeping your head on a swivel and staying aware of your surroundings).
- Playact. The criminal in the above case assumed the women were alone, and he was right. He didn't fear a dog being in the home because they kept running back and forth, and most pooches will want to come outside to see what all the fuss is about. Even if they didn't have a dog, they could have thrown the criminal off by saying something like, "Stay! Be a good boy!" and then casually mentioning to their roommate (so that anyone eavesdropping could overhear), "We don't need our pit bull attacking another person this week!" Something as simple as this could give a criminal pause, especially if they think they know what the status is inside. He could have been watching their place for a while and felt he had pretty good information. Other innocent playacting could be, "Don't mind us, fellas. We'll keep unloading the car while you keep

watching MMA." Another one could be to pretend to talk on the phone as you approach your door, saying something like, "Oh, you and the fellas are just around the corner? OK, see you in a bit!" The sky is the limit on playacting and pretending scenarios that could give a bad person reason to move on. This might sound silly, but remember: most (if not all) criminals want as few challenges to face as possible when they're carrying out their criminal acts. If any doubt can be injected to give them reason to move on, then the strategy is well played. The challenge to this is that you might never know if or when it's worked, so there could be false logic to bail on this tactic because you've never been attacked, not knowing that what you said had saved you from a random act of violence at an unknown place and time.

- Go grocery shopping when you have company over or when you're expecting company. This serves multiple purposes, as you can imagine: more people for a criminal to have to contend with, and more help for you when unloading your goods.

## ✚ Bonus:

For To the Casa, and as a teaser for Chapter 51: Reverse Engineer, instead of assuming someone is following you, you'll intentionally follow someone else. I don't think I need to explain why developing this set of skills can become super valuable, but I will anyway. Yes, of course, in an abduction of a loved one or in a heinous criminal act, following bad guys can help you be able to direct authorities to their whereabouts so they don't get away red-handed (this is likely what comes top of mind, like in the Hollywood high-speed chases). This is a good scenario to contemplate and to train for mentally and physically. However, know that in this scenario the bad guys will be watching their 6 o'clock position to see if anyone is tailing them, and they will cause wrecks, run red lights, and even shoot back to dissuade pursuit. This becomes a great threat to the public, and a lot of innocents can be negatively impacted with multiple lives lost and a wake of property damage. Unless you have time and money to burn, or you have an "in" with the owner of a PVOC-type (police vehicle operations course) operation with miles of paved track with multiple vehicles running scenarios to help you develop this skill, the odds are low that you'll get enough saddle time in the driver's seat to get great at this skill. I'm *not* saying you shouldn't attend specialized driving trainings that these businesses offer; in fact, I highly suggest you make the time and develop a training budget to build skills of this nature and add them to your personal skills package as a responsible citizen. However, it's likely not something you'll be able to practice randomly throughout the week if you read this chapter to then try and execute the following week. And for my last point on these sexy stunt-driving skills courses, they must be done in a controlled environment, and just like in shooting ranges and courses, none of us ever truly know how we will react in certain situations while experiencing real stress in real-life scenarios if they were to play out "live." Multiple chapters are built into this book to support and stack your abilities that create, sharpen, hone, and enhance skills never before experienced to up your (or someone else's) chance for survival. Remember what I said about it being better to have something and not need it than to need it and not have it? Certainly, this is also true in the case of high-pursuit driving, but know that there are so many variables involving so many other drivers, pedestrians, the general public, etc. that we can never plan for how others will react in SHTF scenarios, and no two situations will ever be the same. Knowing you're behind the eight ball and at a disadvantage from the get-go, and driving accordingly, is a wise mental step when pursuing this skill development.

The good news is that there are many other scenarios where tailing someone would be a great set of skills to have to see where someone is going and what they're up to, and to perhaps uncover potential motives, gather further intel, or simply follow at a distance until it is determined they are likely no longer a threat.

There is a great opportunity to practice this skill when you are actually following someone from point A to point B. "Hey, follow me to my cousin's place. We'll fill up the cooler and then head to the lake from there." It's always wise to get the address you're following them to before you set off (if you don't know where point B is), just in case you get separated. In a perfect world, before heading out for the unknown plan B destination, you would plug the coordinates into you GPS, scan the route to have a general idea of where you're going beforehand, and have the navigation as a backup in case you get separated. Otherwise, tail them without the aid of a computer, tablet, smartphone, or navigational app.

## Extra Bonus:

A good progression for the bonus exercise is to purposefully follow someone who knows you're following them. Try to stay behind them at a safe distance, with your vehicle directly behind theirs, one to two cars back. Leaving a space of one to two cars will inevitably happen when other drivers with their own priorities—coupled with their poor, inconvenient, and rude driving skills—cut you off and force their car between you and the vehicle you're following. This weekly exercise can be controlled or uncontrolled. Examples would be a family member, roommate, or friend leaving the house to run an errand. Tell them not to tell you where they are heading, and try to successfully follow them to their destination.

The next progression would be to follow someone who knows they are being followed, and keep a distance where they can't see you following them until you roll up to their destination rendezvous. I love this as a follow-up to the first progression. My wife and I were recently following family members on a vacation to Kanas City and we made sure to follow them far enough back that, during the trip, my wife's aunt called us on two occasions to ask if we were lost or if we were still following them. *Shazam!* Success for one former law enforcement office named Matt Patrick Kelly.

The next progression would be to follow a family member, roommate, or friend without them knowing you're following them, while also trying to elude detection that they are being followed by you.

The final progression would be to follow a random person you've chosen to follow at a distance. *Warning!* Get some skills and develop them in the early stages of this progressive skill-building set. The reason for this is because, when following random unknown folks, if they pick up that you're following them, and they don't know your mission, purpose, or motives, things could escalate rapidly and you might have a situationally aware, protective father who is taking his daughter to gymnastics and sees this unknown vehicle tailing him into the parking lot as a viable threat! With that being said, I absolutely stand behind this progression of skill development, so this step should be taken seriously and pulled off in a manner where you likely won't be detected. This is a more true-to-life execution of this skill. For example, you see a sketchy van trolling your neighborhood streets; they could be casing houses for later burglary or home invasion targets, looking for youth to snag for sinister human trafficking purposes, or any number of other heinous reasons. Following without them knowing they are being followed is a great skill to have and execute at a moment's notice.

Here are some things to consider with the final progression:

- Do this *alone*! Or do it *without* family innocents in the car with you. You don't want a paranoid person picking up your tail and some unpredictable response happens where they double back, turn around on you, and start racing up to your driver's side window while fishing something out of their waistband area.

- If you aren't alone, then rolling with a partner (or partners) who is dependable, levelheaded, and has your back is a good option. If you've all picked this day to train in this exercise together, you can rotate drivers, give positive feedback, etc. Just know that the more people you have in a vehicle trailing someone, the more it looks threatening if you get "made."
- Don't follow people to a final destination. While you're developing this skill, some people might already be good at this, can pick up vibes, and will get a sense for being followed, and now you're on someone's radar, and rightly so.
- Don't follow folks into sketchy areas or neighborhoods. Some really smart people will lead a tail into a place where they have the advantage (such as a pinch point, a dead end, or a place they can exit with great points of cover), leaving the tailing car and all its occupants out in the open and vulnerable for a hail of bullets, thrown rocks/bottles, or a bum-rush from a group of pipe-swinging bikers. Remember, whoever you tail can usually call ahead and give their peeps a heads-up for what to expect when they get to their destination.
- A great way to pull off this last progression is to tail some unknown person for a certain amount of time and/or distance, and then change targets. This way, you're following different people with different skill sets and driving behaviors, and with different sizes, colors, and dimensions of vehicles. Some vehicles and driving patterns are easy to spot and follow while other people (although not necessarily meaning to) are hard as heck to tail and keep eyes on, especially with certain traffic patterns or times of day, such as on suburban streets or in heavy commuter traffic.

## BASIC

# To the Casa

Pretend someone is following you to your house. If you're in a vehicle, scan your mirrors and be aware of what's behind you. Don't go home—this would only show them where you live! Call 911 and go to a police station, firehouse, or busy public place.

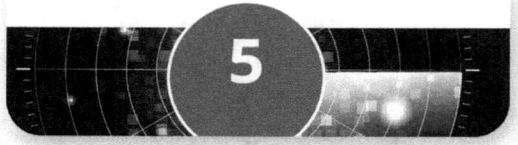

5

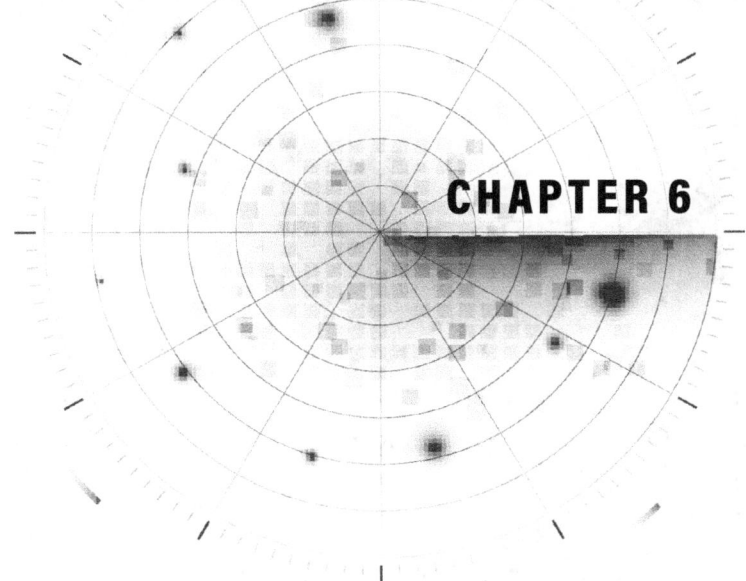

# CHAPTER 6

# RUBBER MEETS THE ROAD

We'll discuss two meanings of this phrase. The first meaning is a personal pulse check, and the second is when driving in stop-and-go traffic.

**Meaning #1:** Where the rubber meets the road is the most important point for something, the moment of truth. An athlete can train all day, but the race is when the rubber meets the road—and when they'll know how good they really are.

**Meaning #2:** When driving, stop far enough behind the vehicle in front of you so that you can see the bottoms of their tires touching the ground, i.e., where the "rubber meets the road."

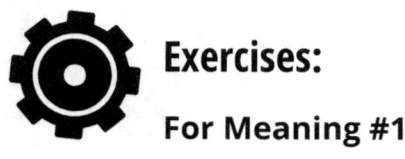

## Exercises:

### For Meaning #1:

If you've followed the chapters in order and have done each for one week (at five days each week), you're a month and a half *in* (25 days of exercises) regarding having situational awareness training under your belt! That's fantastic! You're a trooper, and you should be proud of your efforts to make your safety and the safety of your loved ones a priority! With that being said, it's time to take stock of where you are now, where you were when you began, and how committed you are in making the rest of this work important to you. Has your thinking and thought processes starting to change? Are you starting to look at things and situations differently? Just like in the definition of Meaning #1, regarding the most important point for something, the moment of truth, ask yourself if you are changing, moving forward, and becoming more situationally aware. Ask yourself: How good are you? How good are you willing to become? How committed have you been in executing the exercises so far? How open and committed are you to continuing your personal situational awareness improvement journey? Are they becoming habits or second nature, i.e., something that is becoming part of your personal MOO (method of operation)? This is the moment of truth. You know where you are, you know the efforts you've put forth. If you did some with robust effort and some half-heartedly, now is the time to go back, level set and redrill, then move on. This work is not a race, it's a marathon. And, of course, all exercises can be done randomly or out of order, but as you go through these exercises, the need to reflect on the true meaning of where the rubber meets the road should be considered as a pulse check from time to time as you work to improve your situational awareness. Feel free to set monthly, quarterly, and/or annual check-ins with yourself to reflect on what you've practiced, note improvements, and identify areas and exercises that might be opportunities to revisit and redrill.

## For Meaning #2:

If you operate a motor vehicle on any level of frequency, as you drive—especially in stop-and-go traffic, parking lots, and drive-throughs—stop short of any vehicle that is stopped in front of you so that you can see the bottoms of their rear tires touching the pavement.

The three reasons for this are:

1. If the vehicle in front of you stalls or breaks down, stopping this far back should allow you enough room to pull around them.
2. If you're on a hill and they're operating a manual transmission, they might roll back a bit before moving forward. If your right on their rear end, you could get a lovely "bumper kiss."
3. If you're stopped right on their rear end and the car behind you is stopped on your rear end, you've effectively trapped yourself. This is a situation you don't want to be in if you hear a gunshot, if you see a robbery occurring behind you in the fast-food drive-through lane, or if the vehicle in front of or behind you catches fire. As a driver, you can really only control the distance directly in front of you, and this applies while you're moving and when you're parked. This can potentially leave you at least one out, and it's not a bad strategy to have in a potential carjacking scenario.

## Things to Consider:

In drive-throughs, outside bank teller lanes, etc., give yourself an out. Don't park so close to the car in front of you; instead, try to position your vehicle so that if someone ran up to your door to open it or smash in your driver's side window to carjack you, you'll have a go-to to skedaddle on out of there.

Lock your doors, keep your windows rolled up for as long as possible, use your mirrors to know what is around you and behind you, and "Vision Quest" it (chapter 43) to get a peripheral, 360-degree field of awareness around you and your vehicle.

Note: If I was a junkie and needed cash, I'd chill around ATMs and I'd time when the cash was going to come out, walk up from behind where the mirrors can't see me (working the blind spots), snag the cash, and go before you could grab it. Look for sketchy peeps in maintenance or landscaping shirts and reflective vests. I've seen this crap at Goodwill all day long, and it can give the impression that someone is doing work and has a legit reason for being there, but they can be a criminal who's just trying to blend in. Anyone can buy a reflective high-viz vest at Walmart, Lowe's, or Home Depot. I recently worked a case, in my role as a safety manager, where a guy was walking around in the parking lot of a private, gated retirement community while wearing a reflective vest and pretending to pick up trash. In fact, he was there to steal one of my company's vehicles. Of course, our employee didn't make it hard for the criminal to fulfill his task; it was summertime in Texas, and he'd left his truck running because: 1) It's superhot outside, and who wants to turn off their truck to have it warm by a few degrees when they reenter? 2) No one had ever stolen his truck before, so what were the odds? (Complacency.) 3) It was only a quick drop-off and then he'd be back to the truck. (What could happen?) 4) It's a gated community, so they're safe, right? 5) The "maintenance guy" picking up trash seemed legit.

## BASIC

### Rubber Meets the Road

Whether in stop-and-go traffic or a drive-through lane, if you pull too close and someone does the same behind you, you're trapped. Give yourself room to pull forward and around any vehicles in front of you. Also think about outs, i.e., places you could move toward if you had to.

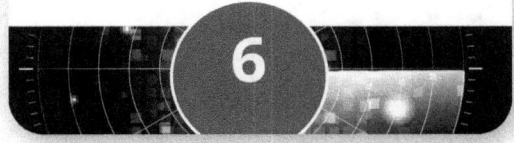

6

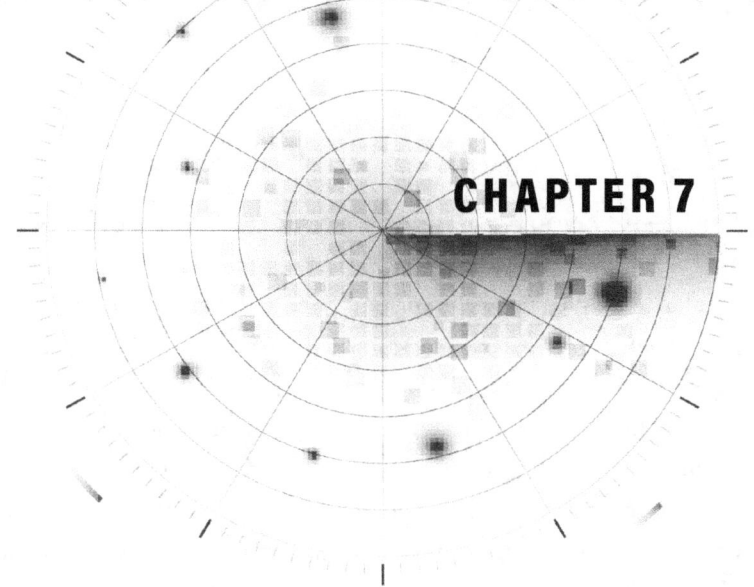

# CHAPTER 7

# PARK SMART

**T**hink about your exit upon your arrival. Back into spots so you can motor away with the best visibility the vehicle was designed to operate in, which is—*duh*—forward!

## Exercise:

Each day this week, park somewhere you wouldn't normally park: farther away, on the side of the building, in the middle of everything, or like Clark Griswold explaining to his boy Rusty why they parked so far away from Wally World when the lot was empty (answer: so they could exit quicker after a day of fun).

## Things to Consider:

What was good and bad about each spot? There will be both—there's not too many "perfect" parking spots in the world—*but* you will start learning and discerning what is better and what is not so smart. So, get good at parking smart. Also, I love the ladies who stay in their car with the doors locked and scan their mirrors to wait for the garage door to close before exiting. You just better make darn sure your mirrors are adjusted to be able to see someone trying to squeeze in before that door squeezes shut. This means you might have to do a wee bit of playing around with the mirror joystick before you pull up into that garage, eh? (I know, this sucks to consider, but if I was a bad dude and I knew you lived alone...the bad guys already think like this.)

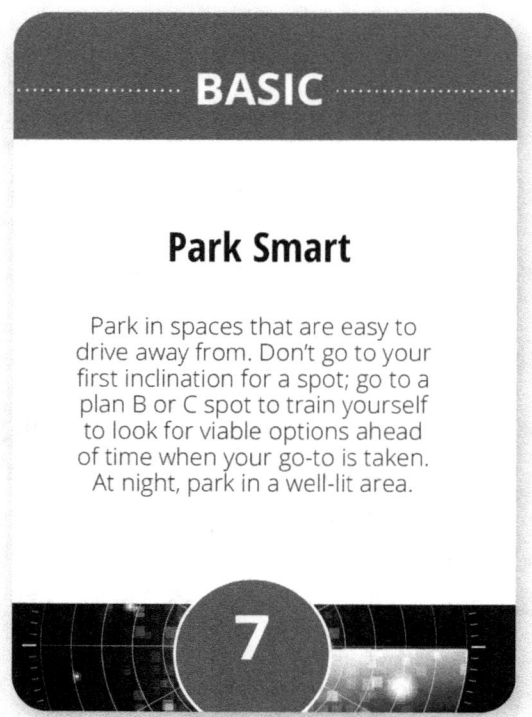

## BASIC

### Park Smart

Park in spaces that are easy to drive away from. Don't go to your first inclination for a spot; go to a plan B or C spot to train yourself to look for viable options ahead of time when your go-to is taken. At night, park in a well-lit area.

7

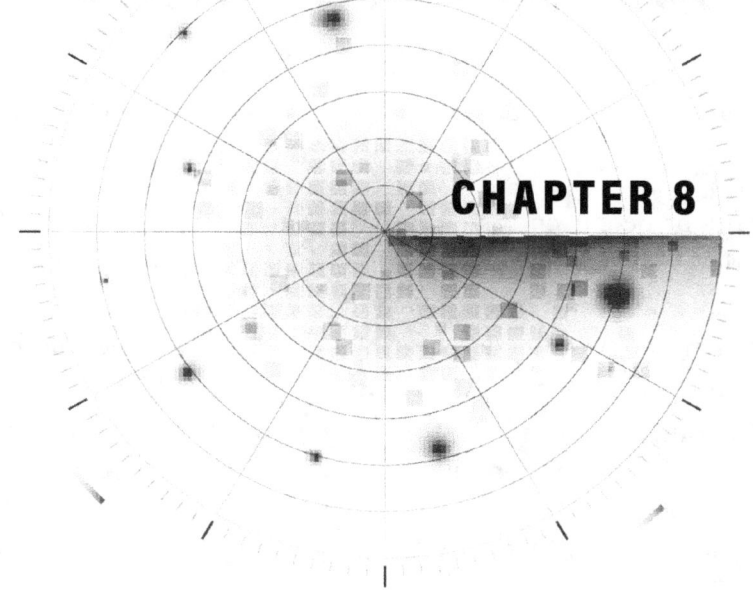

# CHAPTER 8

# BOOK BY ITS COVER

**M**ake a judgment about people based on their appearance.

### Exercise:

Daily throughout the week, look at people and try to size up the toughs and loners, especially those who don't seem to want to be noticed. Who's dangerous? Who seems trustworthy? Who looks like they can handle themselves?

### Things to Consider:

We've had it hammered into us socially to *not* judge a book by its cover. We're told not to judge people by their appearance alone because we don't know their story, past traumas, what they might be currently working through in their lives, etc. *But*, oftentimes, people *do* wear clothing that *screams out* to us and gives us some insights into their character. If it's not clothing and wardrobe, then the face they're "wearing," coupled with their body language, can speak volumes. As in Case the Joint, Odd Man Out, Weapons Inventory, and Vibes, this exercise plays into visual observations, but it also relies on vibes to back up your suspicions. Look at the obvious, but *feel* the room, venue, and/or crowd. Who's trying to play the Gray Man and disappear? Who has the highest likelihood of having road rage, getting on their last nerve, or looking for a fight?

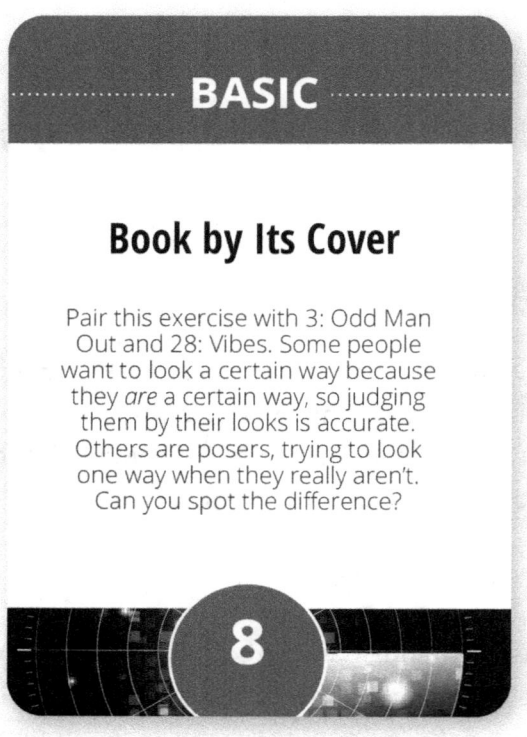

## BASIC

### Book by Its Cover

Pair this exercise with 3: Odd Man Out and 28: Vibes. Some people want to look a certain way because they *are* a certain way, so judging them by their looks is accurate. Others are posers, trying to look one way when they really aren't. Can you spot the difference?

8

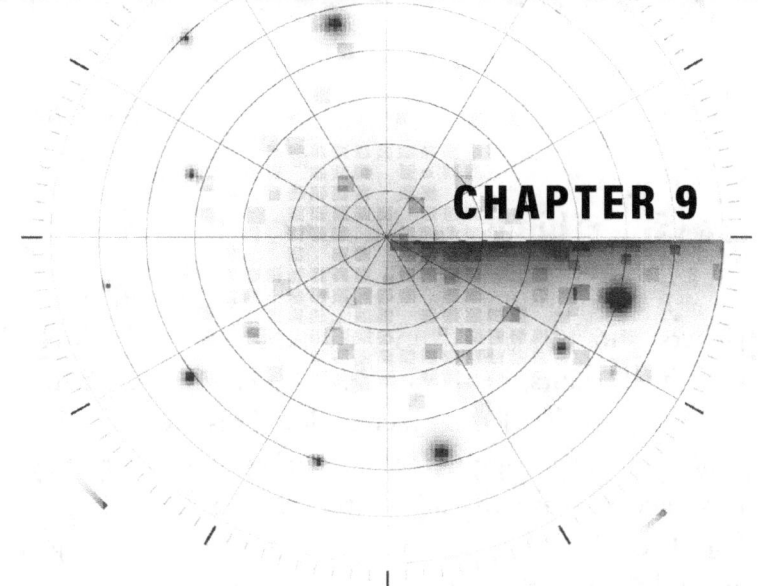

# CHAPTER 9

# HEIGHT AND HAIR COLOR

G et good at getting descriptions of people.

## Exercise:

Each day this week, pick several random people, or folks who give you the heebie-jeebies, and get good at describing them in your mind. Look for more than just their height and hair color, but also take notice of standout features (such as a scar on their nose), their clothing, a ball cap they might be wearing, etc. Give yourself five seconds to get the details, then look away and record your observations. Give yourself more time if needed, and then start dwindling down the time to take in more and more details in a shorter and shorter amount of time.

## Things to Consider:

Although some things can be ditched, such as overshirts, jackets, and ball caps, things that can't be easily ditched are often our shoes, pants, belt, wallet with a chain, etc. (Yup! We gotcha, you wannabe hardcore biker dude!) I also love the hood rats who sport the "sexy" saggin' look. Underwear—which they clearly love to showcase—usually isn't an item that can or will be easily ditched. (Black Under Armour boxer briefs with red lettering and a border around the waistband? Yup! Gotcha, you saggy pant-wearing hood rat!) It's also hard to run like hell and evade arrest when your inseam is down around your knees and you're trying to pull your belt up to your waistline with one hand. It's like chasing waddling penguins, and I'm proud to say I've never lost a footrace to one of these ever-present urban creatures.

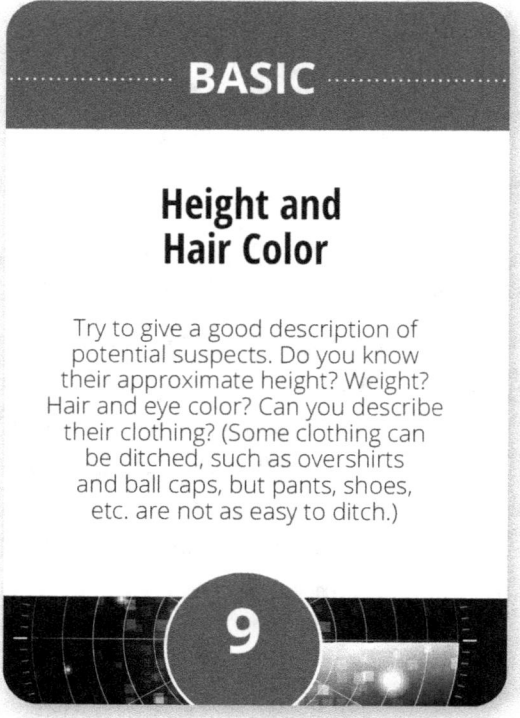

## BASIC

### Height and Hair Color

Try to give a good description of potential suspects. Do you know their approximate height? Weight? Hair and eye color? Can you describe their clothing? (Some clothing can be ditched, such as overshirts and ball caps, but pants, shoes, etc. are not as easy to ditch.)

9

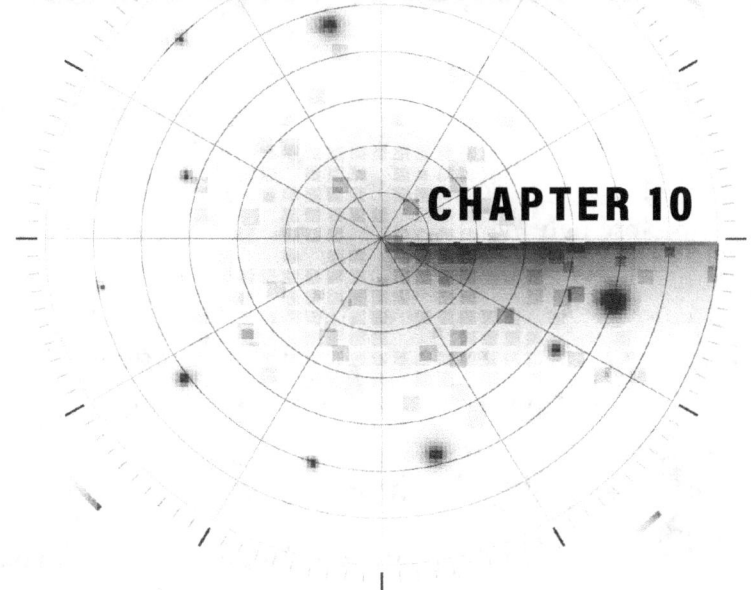

# CHAPTER 10

# ELEVATORS AND STAIRWELLS

**A**re you going alone or with people? Is anyone watching you head to that stairwell door before you head down to the parking garage? You better know!

## ⚙ Exercise:

Each day this week, wherever you find yourself using an elevator or a stairwell, think about times and situations when it would be favorable and when it would be unfavorable. A crowd in a stairwell might be a great thing when you're heading down to the parking garage after the office closes, but perhaps not so great when you're sharing it with a bunch of drunken soccer-fan hooligans. If you're the last one to leave the office late at night, taking those stairs or jumping on that elevator might not be the wisest thing to do. An elevator is a box, a larger version of the phone booth relic, it's like a tiny boxing ring with walls. The point is, unless you're great at up-close fighting and an expert at keeping your head from being bounced off of walls, blocking knees to the body/groin, and fending off elbows to the face, your space is limited in this environment. Figure out times, schedules, and multiple options. There is usually more than one stairwell or elevator in a building.

## Things to Consider:

If I was a bad guy and I wanted to attack you in a stairwell, I'd want to use gravity to assist me. I could attack from the high ground, above you, and let the hard corners and edges of the stairs do some work for me as you fell backward. I could grab you from behind, pulling you backward and letting the walls, handrails, and stair edges help me do some damage to you as well. See Chapter 18: Hair Is a Handle for some details on grab points. Regarding elevators, we all seem to get shy and want to "disappear" when we're in a confined space with a bunch of strangers. Be sure and Back It Up, Back It In (from chapter 27) so you have your back against the wall. This isn't easy to do if you're the last one on a crowded elevator, but I'd rather have my back to the closing doors facing the unknown crowds (making them uncomfortable) versus me being uncomfortable and exposing my back to the unknown within the tight space of an elevator. You could also Get Sideways (chapter 26), or just wait for another elevator or take the stairs. When you're in an elevator, you are trapped inside a small, four-walled space, even if for a short time (if it's working properly and you don't get stuck in one). For you New Yorkers and other big-city dwellers, this becomes a monumental exercise, and you could also throw in subways and buses to have plenty of homework to do. Your options are limited, and likely you'll be sharing some paths of travel that are undesirable. Luckily, this book has multiple chapters and exercises for you to stack and build good habits upon. Study all the chapters and perform the weekly exercises to raise your situational awareness in these super busy, crowded environments.

The last thing to consider is to try being on an elevator with multiple people you trust. Multiple people mean multiple witnesses to a bad person. Especially helpful would be a companion who knows how to protect themselves and others. (I'd certainly feel more comfortable and at ease during the trip between floors!)

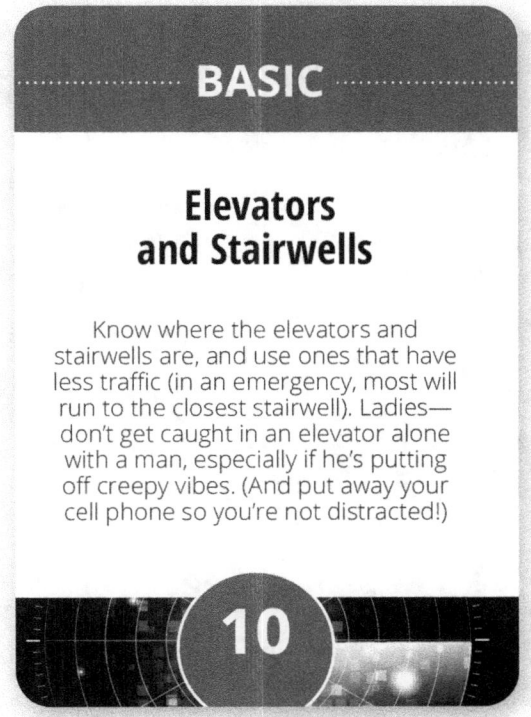

**BASIC**

### Elevators and Stairwells

Know where the elevators and stairwells are, and use ones that have less traffic (in an emergency, most will run to the closest stairwell). Ladies—don't get caught in an elevator alone with a man, especially if he's putting off creepy vibes. (And put away your cell phone so you're not distracted!)

10

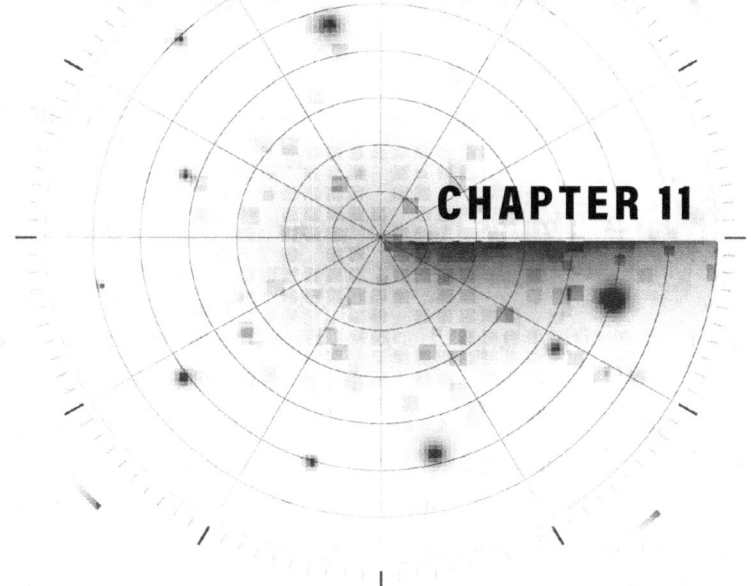

# CHAPTER 11

# SHOES ARE CLUES

I f I told you that you'd have to run for your life today, would you wear those five-inch stilettos to work today? What people choose to put on their feet are telltale signs of what they expect out of their day, which is usually nothing unexpected or out of the ordinary. I love airports for this because so many flip-flops, sandals, and Crocs would come flying off of people's feet as they scattered to flee across ground that could potentially be covered in broken glass that had been shattered by an angry guy with a machine gun.

## Exercise:

Wear only functional footwear for the week. If possible, aim to select footwear that is multifunctional for multiple environments and surfaces. Wear footwear that would support you running for your life, if you had to.

## Things to Consider:

You might have some new camping boots hidden away in a shoebox, waiting for an upcoming trip. Break these in now versus cutting blisters while you're out in the bush. If you have multiple shoes and/or boots that fulfill this week's exercise, then wear a different pair each day of the week. You might discover that some are better than others, and some might be better suited for specific environments than you might have thought (like on wet or slick sidewalks). I'm a big fan of shoes and boots that lace up over the ankle. Rolling an ankle could severely hamper your ability to skedaddle away from someone or something.

## Bonus:

You might discover that you need to go shopping! *But* do your research and read some reviews!

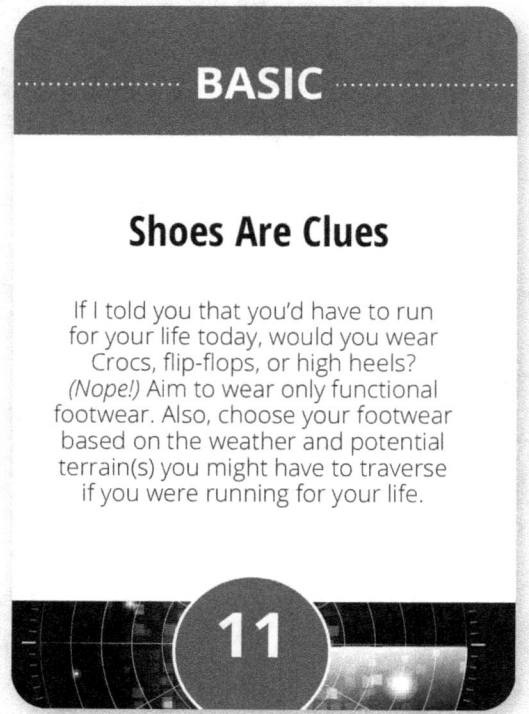

### BASIC

### Shoes Are Clues

If I told you that you'd have to run for your life today, would you wear Crocs, flip-flops, or high heels? *(Nope!)* Aim to wear only functional footwear. Also, choose your footwear based on the weather and potential terrain(s) you might have to traverse if you were running for your life.

**11**

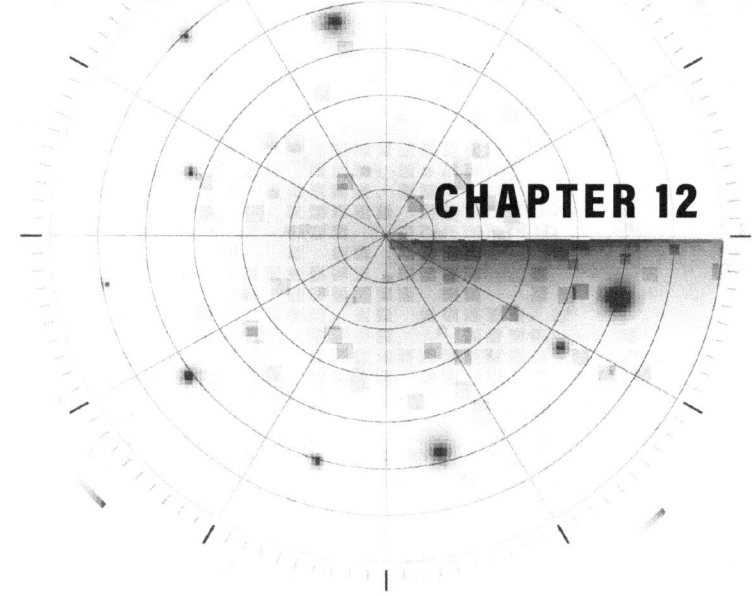

# CHAPTER 12

# KNOW THE NUMBERS

**M**emorize phone numbers and addresses that are important to you. If you don't, you're just being lazy! Phones break and wallets with notes, cards, and other information can get stolen or lost (i.e., when you're running for your life), and there is always the unexpected car wreck that can cause personal belongings to get broken or become misplaced.

## Exercise:

Each day this week, pick at least one important phone number to memorize. If that person doesn't live with you, memorize their address as well. This exercise might bleed into other weekly memorization homework if you have more than five to seven key peeps you love and want to help and protect if the need calls for it. Then, knowing their description (height, weight, hair color, eye color, etc.), as well as vehicle(s) they might own, drive, or use, and their work address, would be beneficial brainwork to add onto this week's memory work.

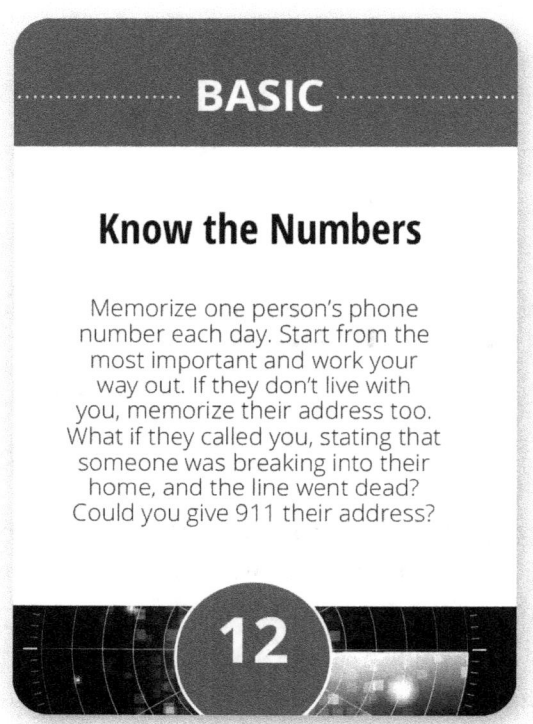

**BASIC**

## Know the Numbers

Memorize one person's phone number each day. Start from the most important and work your way out. If they don't live with you, memorize their address too. What if they called you, stating that someone was breaking into their home, and the line went dead? Could you give 911 their address?

**12**

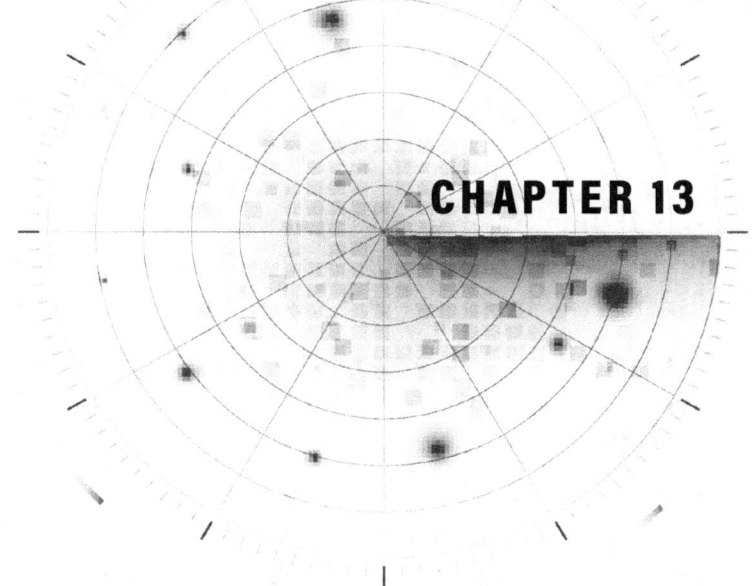

# KNOW YOUR LIMITS

This means your home or work location is your "ground zero" or starting point.

## ⚙ Exercise:

From your home, think of your neighbors, from those closest in to those farthest out. Then think of your family, friends, and acquaintances from there. These are your tiers of go-tos in a bugout scenario. These can also become your layers of warning if/ as things come to you. If you don't know your neighbors (at home or at work), then it's a good idea to introduce yourself and get on some level of familiarity with them. Offering a compliment, asking for a small favor, or giving a favor can go a long way in beginning a trusting relationship; plus, it's the neighborly thing to do! Each day, work from closest to your house/work location outward.

**Day 1:** Think of all the places that you can walk to from your home/ground zero. Who could you go to, and who might listen to you and allow you access to their environment?

**Day 2:** Think of all the places that you could drive to from your home/ground zero. Who could you go to, and who might listen to you and allow you access to their environment?

**Day 3:** Think of all the places that you can walk to from your work/ground zero. Who could you go to, and who might listen to you and allow you access to their environment?

**Day 4:** Think of all the places that you could drive to from your work/ground zero. Who could you go to, and who might listen to you and allow you access to their environment?

**Day 5:** Do the exercises from days 1–4 based on being somewhere else, such as on your latest vacation, on a future vacation, at a family member's home, etc.

By performing these exercises, you are identifying tiers and layers of offense, defense, and communication. It goes from in to out, and from out to in.

## Things to Consider:

Mapping these things and having them marked via a computer, a phone, and a GPS system—as well as a physical paper map—are all going to support you in this week's exercises. This is a great exercise to combine with Chapter 20: Gather and Then Go.

### BASIC

## Know Your Limits

Know your friends, family, and
acquaintances who live near you,
from closest to farthest away. They
are your perimeters of go-tos. In
a bugout situation, who could you
reasonably walk or drive to that
would take you in? Who would you
take in if the roles were reversed?

13

# INTERMEDIATE

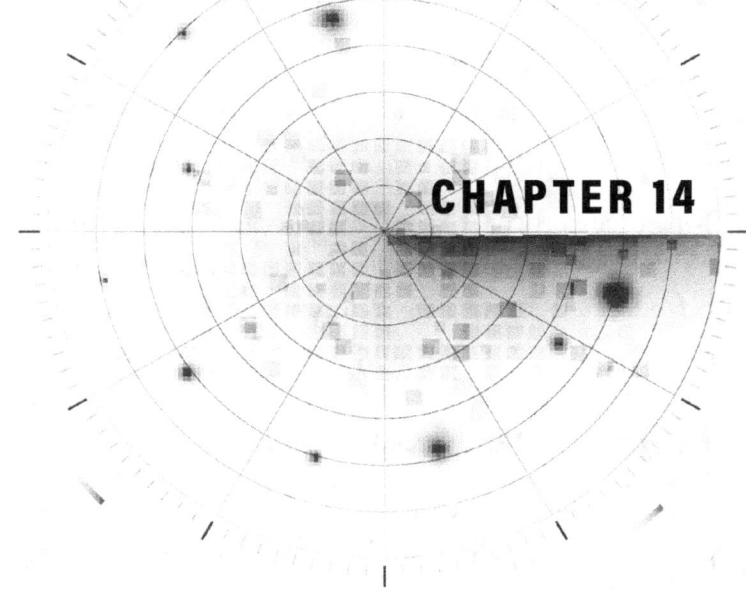

# BLUE FOUR-DOOR SEDAN WITH TEXAS PLATES

This is a piggyback off of Chapter 5: To the Casa. Add this to the exercises in chapters 4 and 5, or do it on its own.

## Exercise:

Do this exercise for at least five days throughout the week. Assuming no one is actually following you home, when you reach the end of your driveway (or as you turn into your apartment complex, reach your gate to enter the entry code, etc.) make note of the next vehicle that passes by and get a description of it. It's description *and* occupants/number of occupants can be important. If there are multiple occupants, that's better intel than a description of a solo driver. Don't get bogged down in the details. As a former law enforcement officer, I know that having a basic vehicle description with the number of occupants is usually plenty to give the police probable cause to pull over a potential recalcitrant group and determine what nonsense they might have been up to.

## Things to Consider:

Make note of the color of the vehicle, number of doors, type (i.e. sedan, pickup, SUV), foreign (Kia, Toyota, Honda) or domestic (Chevy, Ford, Dodge), and make/model (Ford Taurus). These are all great identifiers, along with the number of occupants (driver with two passengers in the back). Here's an example: Black four-door Ford pickup with two passengers in the front. It's good to get the order "baked" in your mind now versus having to think about it in a stressful situation. My cadence is color, number of doors, make, model, and occupants. If I don't know the make and model, one or the other is decent, or knowing whether it's a foreign or domestic make. As you practice, your brain will start taking in these details in the order you've chosen. Also, as you get good with the exercises in Chapter 5: To the Casa, you can start picking up these details and descriptions as someone is tailing you, especially when you make turns. The lighting might not be optimal, or it could be at night, or when it's storming or raining, so timing your mirror spots rearward as you pass streetlights (especially streetlights at corners) is a good strategy to keep in mind. Finally, this doesn't have to be done only when you're heading home. This exercise can be done when you're going anywhere: to the store, to the movies, on road trips, etc. This can also be done while you're stationary. For example, you're at a park, enjoying a picnic. Practice getting a description of the car that just went by, especially if it goes by more than once, whereby your doggone Spidey sense better be sounding off situational awareness warning bells in your head!

## + Bonus:

If you can get the state of the license plate and a couple of digits or letters, even better! This is a great skill to develop, but all skills are perishable if you don't practice them and keep them honed. Should you ever truly have to call 911 and give a decent description of what Johnny Law should look for, this skill can mean the difference between someone getting caught—and caught quickly—or getting away to terrorize another person (or, God forbid, you on a later day). This takes time and practice, but you can get excellent at it as time goes on. Popping out your phone and making a voice memo or a recording, or saying the description over and over out loud or silently in your head until you potentially have to make the 911 call, will help your short-term memory as you can forget vital info when the 911 operator asks questions. Hint: when you hear "911, what's your emergency?" spout out as the first words out of your mouth the description as clearly and calmly as possible. Your location, the reason for the call, and other details will be determined as the call goes on. FYI: 911 operators are some of the *most* amazing human beings on the planet! They bust the myth of multitasking and are sending out info as they gather it, and either they or another operator are dispatching this information through an MDT (mobile dispatch terminal) or live via another operator. Having that vehicle description from the get-go is *awesomeness*. Your location would be the next logical question, followed by why you're calling.

### Extra Bonus:

This is a good game to play with a friend, on a family road trip, etc. For example: "That brown vehicle that just exited—tell me what you can about it." Another could be, after a restroom break during a road trip, to ask questions like: "While we were in the convenience store, how many people were in there? How many men? How many women? Did you see the sketchy dude with the camo pants who noticed you walk to the bathroom? What can you tell me about his description?" OK, that last one might not be such a fun-time bonus exercise, and you could scare the crap outta some of the people you're with, but this skill is invaluable. I *make sure* if the "sketchy camo dude" thing happens in real life (and it has), for example, if I'm at a store and my wife or daughter are eyed anywhere in the store or when walking to or from the ladies' room, that the camo dude *knows* I *saw him* and that I saw him seeing them. They usually slink away and try to hide or blend in...which is somewhat hard to do with a fella like me around!

## Bonus Things to Consider:

Don't be a Nazi, we-gotta-make-good-time kind of traveler. Make a plan, and then execute to the plan. You don't need to gas up the car while your loved ones go inside, only to have them exit and sit in the car while you take your potty break, leaving them alone and unprotected in the car with it *running* while the AC is kicked on high so the road trip can continue to be a joy. Go as a group! Walk in together, get your business taken care of together, and exit together. Everyone can wait an extra five minutes with the windows rolled down while you pump go-juice into the family truckster before getting back on your way to see the largest ball of yarn in America. Be smart! I believe in you!

## INTERMEDIATE

# Blue Four-Door Sedan with Texas Plates

If someone was following you in a vehicle or drove by your location and did something criminal, could you get a decent description? For the next vehicle that passes you, practice this skill. Have a go-to order (ex: color, number of doors, make and model, state plate, and number of occupants).

14

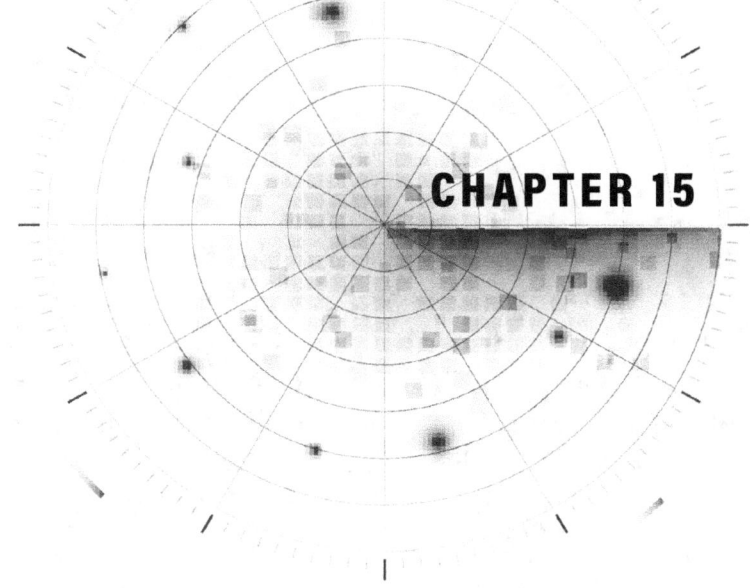

# CHAPTER 15

# CASE THE JOINT

I f you don't know, then don't go. Assumptions can get you in trouble, so be wise by taking in information that can validate or invalidate actions you want to take.

## Exercise:

Each day this week, before you exit your vehicle and enter any business, store, or public building, "case the joint"—like the criminals do.

## Things to Consider:

When pulling up to a convenience store, look for people who are still in their vehicles before exiting your vehicle. Also look for people who are standing around, trying to look inconspicuous. For example, if it's summertime in Texas and I see a dude go in the store wearing a bulky jacket with the hood pulled up, I'm not going in. If you see five dudes chillin' in an old beater van with paper license plate tags, paying attention to all of the people coming and going in and out of that store, don't go in. Instead, chill, watch, and wait. Count cars and heads before you enter. If there are nine cars in the lot and you can't see any people moving around inside, there might be an armed robbery happening back in the cooler and you could be walking into an undesirable situation.

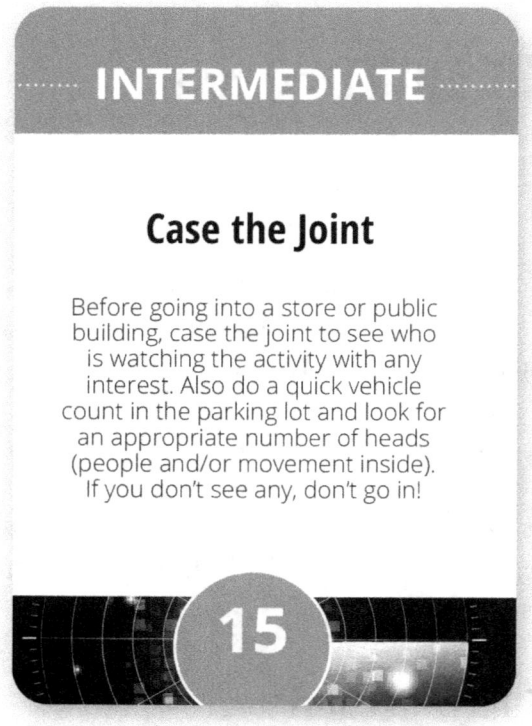

## INTERMEDIATE

### Case the Joint

Before going into a store or public building, case the joint to see who is watching the activity with any interest. Also do a quick vehicle count in the parking lot and look for an appropriate number of heads (people and/or movement inside). If you don't see any, don't go in!

**15**

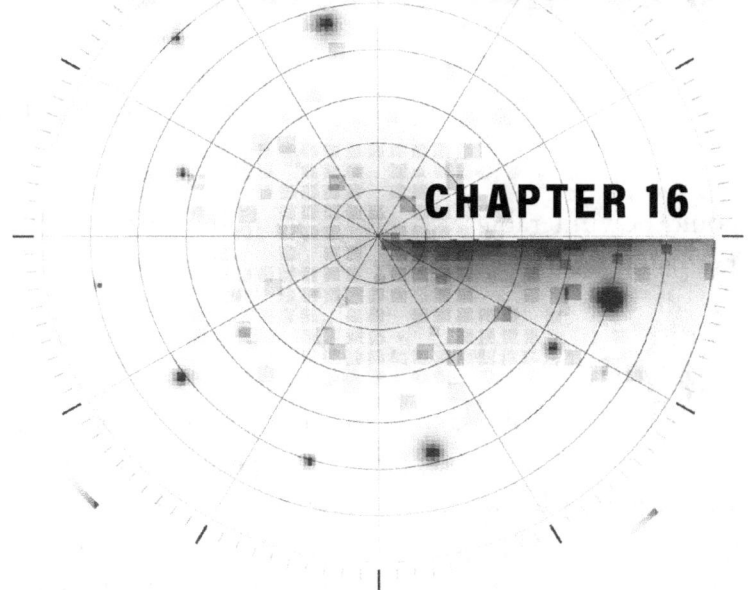

# CHAPTER 16

# OUT OF TOUCH

Keep yourself out of easy reach. Just like with Chapter 41: Tag, You're It, if someone were to try to tag you, can they snag instead of tag? A purse, a cell phone, your wallet, your Uncle Mike's OWB holstered *pistola* with no retention...these are items that could potentially be snagged.

## Exercise:

Like in the exercise for Tag, You're It, during this week's exercise, don't let anyone who isn't a family member, friend, or acquaintance get close enough to snag anything from your person. Do this in every place you visit over the next five days. This means being mindful of what you carry, where you carry it, and when and how you display it (having it out in the open, such as with your cell phone, car keys, or wallet). You might be surprised by habits you've formed regarding what you carry, how you carry it, and when you could be vulnerable to someone grabbing something of yours and taking off with it.

## Things to Consider:

The more stuff you have, the more opportunities there are for something to be potentially snagged and taken. I don't carry anything of value in my back pockets (just a plastic comb and one or two flossers). All my goodies are on the front side of me, from my hip bones to just short of my centerline on both sides. Incorporating other exercises from this book while executing this week's exercise is wise. A few good ones to pile onto this are Chapter 41: Tag You're It, Chapter 27: Back It Up, Back It In, and Chapter 26: Get Sideways.

## INTERMEDIATE

### Out of Touch

Keep your belongings out of reach. Don't pull out your valuables unless it's absolutely necessary (even at ATMs, the bank, and stores). Also, keep only what you absolutely need on your person, and place valuables on you in places that would be hard to pickpocket without you noticing.

16

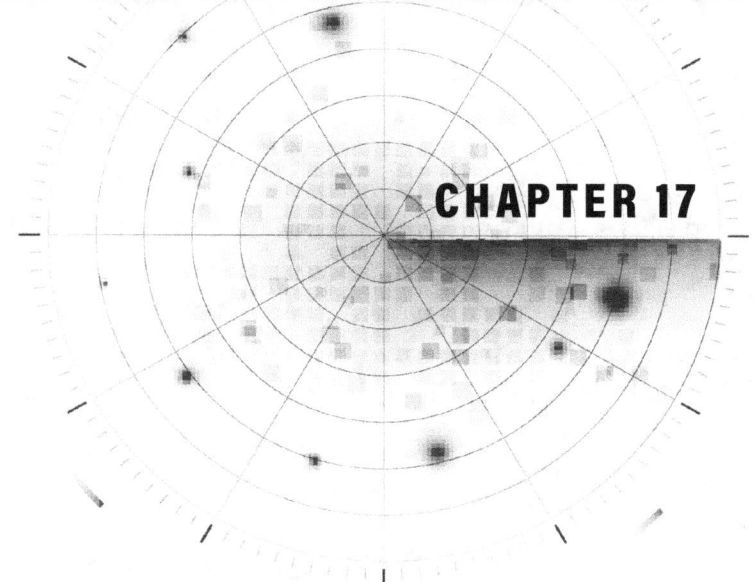

# CHAPTER 17

# FIND A WAY—OR MAKE ONE

**W**hen exits aren't an option, can you make one? Windows? Drywall?

## Exercise:

In multiple places you find yourself in during each day of the week, imagine that the exits are not an option, i.e., that's where the bad guys are standing or where the fire is burning. What other options can you find, discover, and make as viable options to get out of a building?

## Things to Consider:

Do you have a glass-breaker embedded at the end of your pocketknife, tactical pen, or other implements that can get the job done? A heavy chair might do the trick with a couple of hefty swings, but would you have the time in an emergency? Windows may seem easy, but they are often sturdy and designed to withstand severe weather such as hail and high winds. Likewise, windows on vehicles have safety glass and are designed to withstand collisions. Do you know where to hit glass to break it? *Not in the middle!*

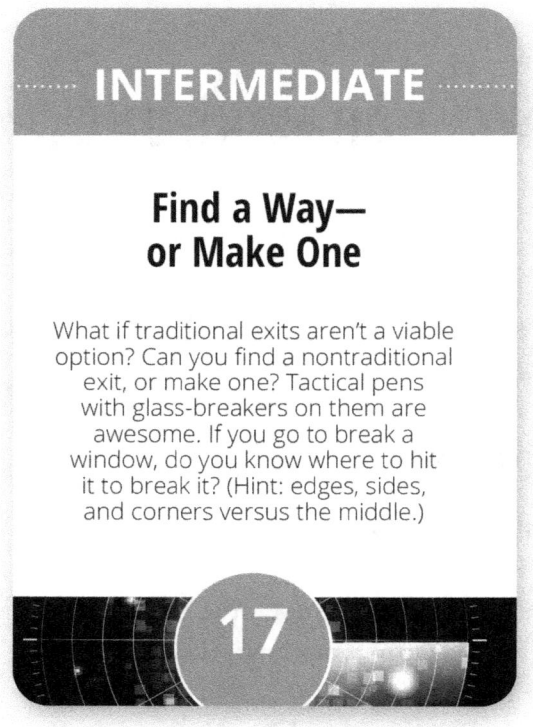

## INTERMEDIATE

### Find a Way— or Make One

What if traditional exits aren't a viable option? Can you find a nontraditional exit, or make one? Tactical pens with glass-breakers on them are awesome. If you go to break a window, do you know where to hit it to break it? (Hint: edges, sides, and corners versus the middle.)

17

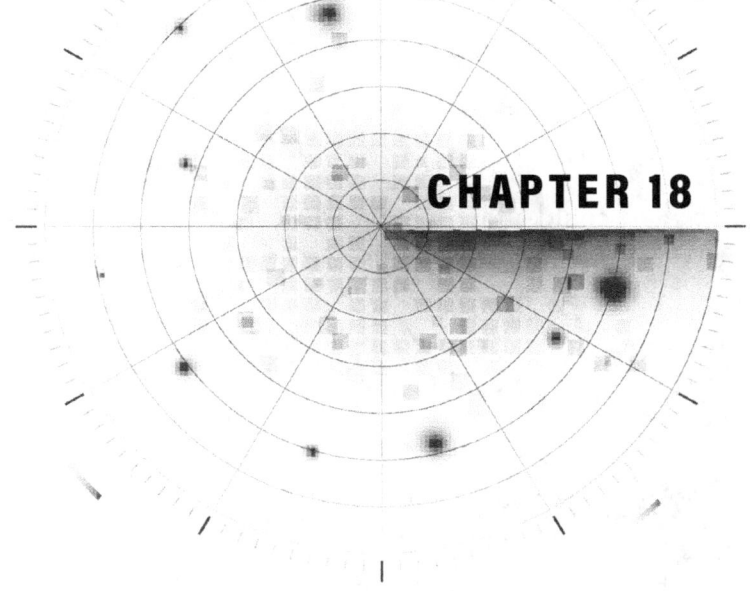

# CHAPTER 18

# HAIR IS A HANDLE

So are hoodies and belts. One of my favorite martial arts principles/techniques I've learned is this: control the head and you control the body. Hair can be a handle, especially if it's long enough to grip and/or it's real hair! My arms and upper body are stronger than most, if not all, necks, and I could likely swizzle-stick you around if I had a good enough handle that was attached to your head.

### Exercise:

Take note of your hair and how it is arranged. I'm not asking you to cut your hair, but you should be aware of this disadvantage and not let people get within tagging distance (see Chapter 41: Tag, You're It). Can you arrange your hair so it's less of a handle? Also, it's important to take stock of clothing you're wearing, such as hoodies, shirts, and jackets that could be great handles around the neck and could allow someone to control your head. This is also a good exercise for those folks with short hair or shaved heads that don't present a great handle. Each day this week, choose a hairstyle and/or wardrobe that isn't as "handle-friendly" around the neck as other choices you could wear. Couple this week's exercise with Tag, You're It.

## Things to Consider:

Belts are great handles, too! A lot of grappling arts such as Brazilian jujitsu and wrestling teach how to control the hips, along with controlling the head, to gain control over opponents. I'm not going to give up my sturdy tactical belt that I wear on the daily, because I need a solid platform for my holster and pistol to be deployed from. I'm not going to swap this out for a "breakaway" belt, because the tactical one creates a fantastic handle. However, I can untuck my shirt over my belt so it becomes harder to detect exactly where it is. Doing this is a solid plan, especially when paired with being situationally aware of my environment with exercises in this book to identify people prior to them getting within arm's reach of grabbing my belt for use as a handle.

Getting training from a qualified instructor, system, school, or dojo in a martial art that suits itself to grappling defenses against hair grabs and hip control (among many other scenarios) is definitely something everyone should consider. Brazilian jujitsu, judo, and wrestling come top of mind when thinking of good places to start. I don't want to piss off a judoka within arm's reach, outside on a chilly day, standing on concrete while wearing a heavy winter jacket!

## INTERMEDIATE

### Hair Is a Handle

Control the head, control the body. Hair can be a handle, and so can collars, hoodies, and belts. If someone gets close enough, they can grab a "handle," so don't let them, and/or wear clothing or hairstyles that don't present as much of a handle as others.

18

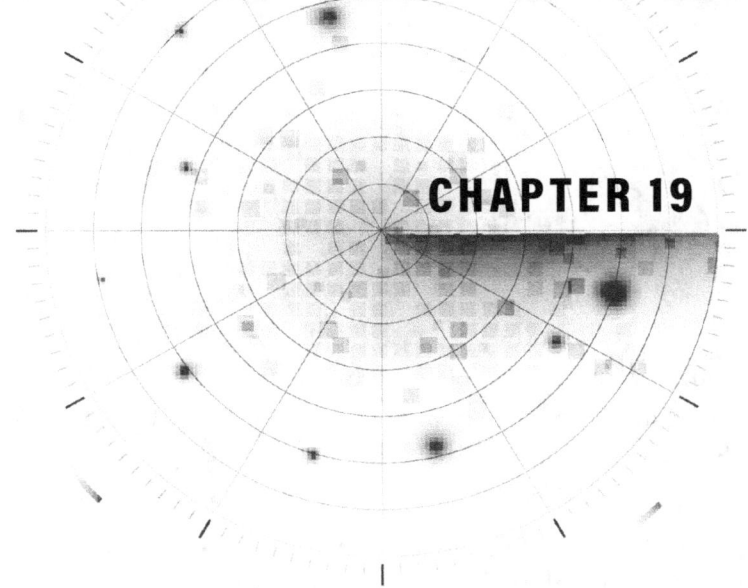

# CHAPTER 19

# WHO'S WITH ME?

**A**re you by yourself or with another/others?

### ⚙ Exercise:

Each day this week, take notice of when you are alone and when you are with another person or persons. If you're alone, this is one scenario where you'd want to contemplate the What-If Game from chapter 48. If you're with a loved one, this creates a different scenario to contemplate, as it would if you were with multiple loved ones. Mentally walk through these scenarios, and if others are open to it, talk through some what-if scenarios with them, too.

## Things to Consider:

Do you have an alert word for a home emergency that lets everyone know where to go and what to do? Do you have a rally point? Whether you're alone or with loved ones, play out where you are at any given time, in the places you find yourself figuring out things such as: "Well, because I'm with my significant other and child, this is the strategy I'd likely use. But if they weren't with me, I'd likely stand over there because..." You come up with your own answers—thinking is free, it doesn't cost a dime. Now is the time to mentally compute and figure it out. Plus, I won't be there with you when the SHTF. And even if I was, I promise you, I have different priorities and reasons to live than you do, so my execution of my actions during a man-made or natural emergency situation could be very different compared to yours.

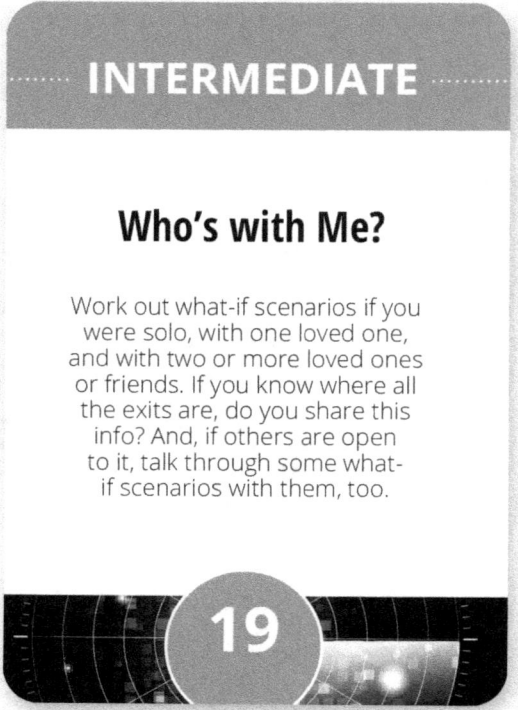

### INTERMEDIATE

### Who's with Me?

Work out what-if scenarios if you were solo, with one loved one, and with two or more loved ones or friends. If you know where all the exits are, do you share this info? And, if others are open to it, talk through some what-if scenarios with them, too.

19

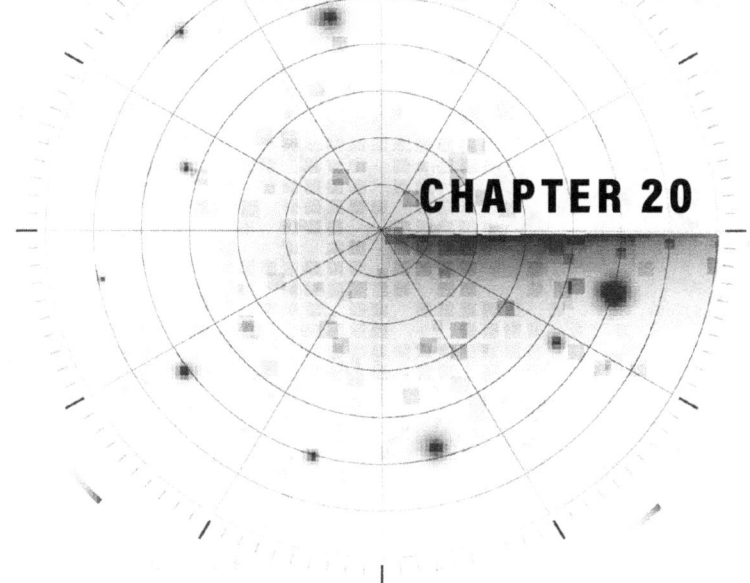

# GATHER AND THEN GO

G et intel before you head downtown to your favorite restaurant. Is there a protest going on and they're burning up hardware stores?

### Exercise:

Each day, before you go somewhere, scan the news, Internet, and happenings to see if anything is "up" before you go. You might be surprised at what you find, even if it's just a local farmers market you didn't know about. (If this is the case, don't waste good intel—go shopping for some healthy food!)

## INTERMEDIATE

# Gather and Then Go

Before heading out, gather intel
to determine if it's a good idea.
You might learn there's a farmers
market next to where you're
going. (Awesome! Shop for fresh
veggies!) Or you might learn there's
a protest happening a block away.
(Might wanna pick a different
place, or stay in altogether!)

20

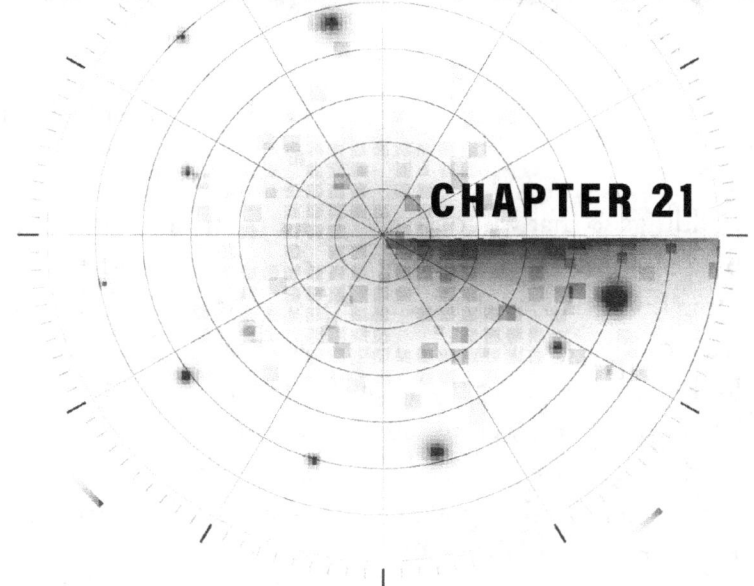

# GET THE BIG PICTURE

This doesn't have to be a 30,000-foot view; make it personal. We live in a 3D world, so think about what's up high, what's down low, what's far away, and what's near. We've discussed close encounters in Tag, You're It (chapter 41), and now you'll also pull in what could be far away that could still negatively affect you, like bullets from a long-range rifle.

## Exercise:

Each day this week, make it a point to be aware three-dimensionally and in a 360-degree sphere around your person, around the persons you're with, and/or in a group of people you're in the company of. This will piggyback with a later chapter, Aim High (chapter 23).

And now for a personal share: When I was a rookie at the Dallas Police Academy, we cadets played both cops and bad guys hiding in buildings so that we could practice answering burglary calls, etc. The biggest sin most of us committed was that our field of vision was often limited to head height and just a few feet in front of us, meaning we would often just scan from eye level to the floor, forgetting to look up. I would get high, low, and cram my body into tight places where most of my classmates didn't think a grown man could hide. I'd then scare the *crud* outta my classmates as they passed my hiding spots when I either grabbed them, poked them, or yelled at them. Hide-and-go-seek pro? Or deviant country boy who used to play "ninja" on neighbors' private property just to see how close to a house I could get without their dogs knowing I was there? I'll let you decide. FYI: knowing wind direction, and what not to step on that could make a crunching sound, were bonuses when trying to elude canine sniffers with superb hearing.

## ✚ Bonus:

If you finally notice that water stain on a ceiling tile above your office desk, you're doing great!

## INTERMEDIATE

# Get the Big Picture

Maintain a 360-degree sphere of awareness around your person, and don't forget to look up, down, and side to side when getting the big picture. This is harder to do in a vehicle, but adjusting your mirrors and turning your head side to side can cut down on blind spots.

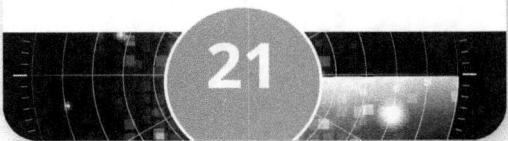

**21**

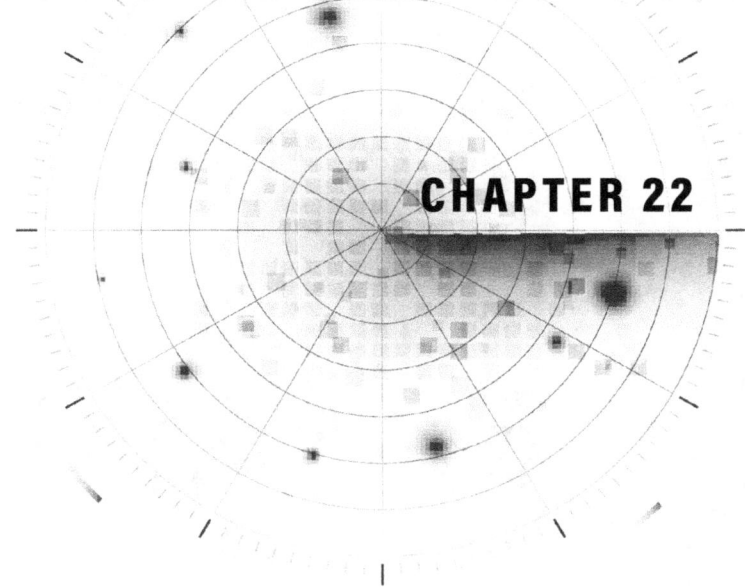

# CHAPTER 22

# ENVIRONMENT

What is the current weather or environment like? How bad is it? Could it get worse? What should you consider taking with you if you had to flee to safety? Are you prepared?

## Exercise:

If your weather is the same most of the time or during this week, pick a day each week to prep for snow, heavy rain, a tornado, an earthquake, civil unrest, etc.

## INTERMEDIATE

# Environment

Prep your personal vehicle with
anything you'd need to have on hand
if you had to flee to safety or deal
with an environmental challenge
such as massive rain and flooding, a
blizzard, an earthquake, a tornado,
extreme heat, or civil unrest.

**22**

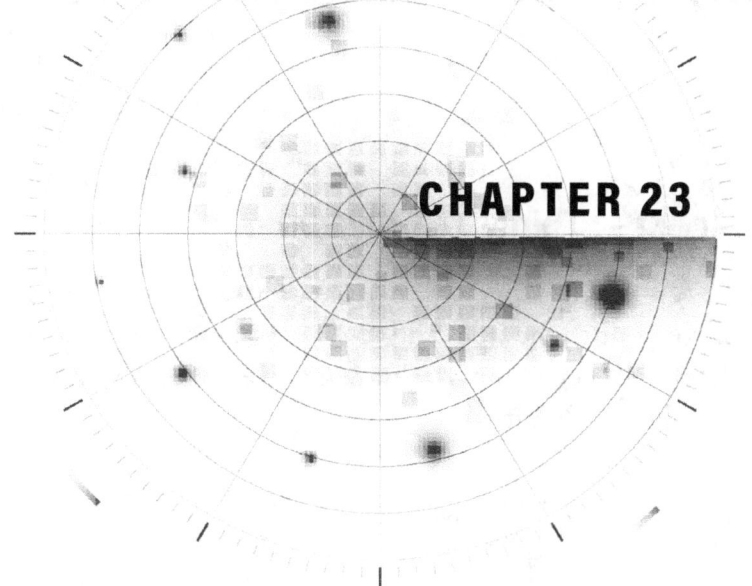

# CHAPTER 23

# AIM HIGH (HORIZON AND BACK)

**E**ye your lead time, from yourself to the horizon and back again.

## Exercise:

Every day this week, or as often as you can remember, visually scan and look as far out as you can. Mentally take in everything you see from the horizon and back to you. Don't do it so fast that you can't take in valuable information. Rinse and repeat. This is known as reading a room, and it will allow you to visually and mentally take note of what's in your environment. Using other exercises from this book, what stands out? Who is trying not to stand out? Are you picking up any vibes from a certain area, spot, group, or person? If so, that might be worth paying attention to and keeping tabs on.

## Things to Consider:

Do this with peripheral vision. Don't just look in front of you, but to the sides and to your 6 o'clock (rear), and don't forget the 3D aspect of our world, which we talked about in Chapter 21: Get the Big Picture.

### Aim High (Horizon and Back)

Similar to the 360-degree sphere of awareness from 39: Get the Big Picture, look out as far as you can (ex: to the horizon), and take in all of the information, from far to near, and back to you. You can also do this to your left, right, and rearward.

23

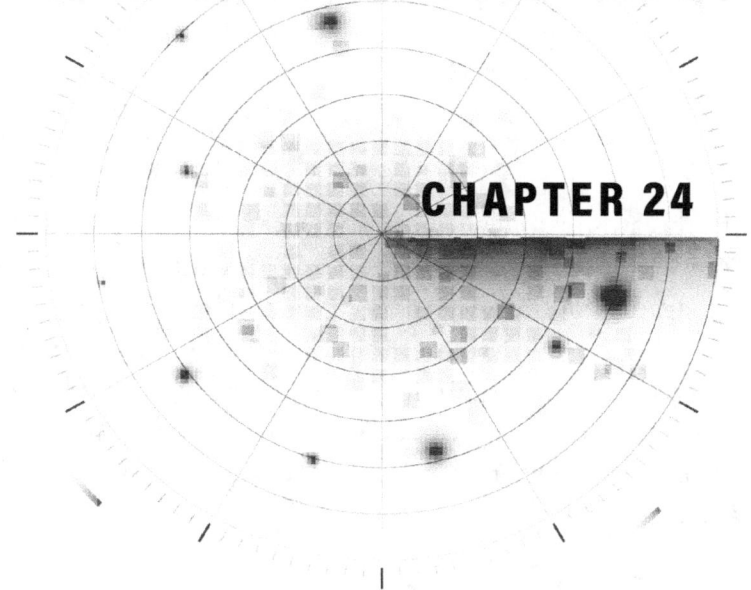

# CHAPTER 24

# *BREATHE!* (IF YOU WANNA LIVE)

**M**ore important to our survival than food and water is the air we breathe. Nothing is more important for our ability to continue living than oxygen! To be the most aware, you need good, oxygenated blood to be moving through your body, especially to your brain, so that you can take in information to make good decisions. How do we get this? By breathing. In our modern-day society, most of us breathe like crap, taking shallow breaths, taking too many breaths, and failing to expel all of the carbon dioxide (dead air) from our lungs, versus getting an oxygenated lungful of Mother Earth's life-giving air.

### Exercise:

Each day this week, perform box breathing (also known as autogenic breathing, or combat or tactical breathing) a minimum of three times. To do box breathing, inhale for four seconds, hold this breath for four seconds, fully exhale for four seconds, and hold "empty" at the bottom of the breath for four seconds before inhaling again for four seconds to start the breathing cycle over again. Do this for a minimum of four cycles at least three times a day (ex: morning, noon, and night). Since I started practiced box breathing, I've graduated from 4x4s to 5x5s and then to doing it by what feels natural and comfortable. I can now take two and a half full breaths and exhalations in one minute.

## Things to Consider:

While inhaling, imagine this in two stages. First, fill up your belly, lower lungs, and diaphragm. Then move up from the bottom of your lungs to the top (I visualize this as filling to my collarbone). I hold this breath for my desired count, then upon exhalation, I visualize my belly, lungs, and windpipe as a bellows, with the tip being my windpipe. As I exhale, I squeeze all the air from my belly, up and out completely through my throat. I pull my abdominal muscles as far in as possible, imagining them squeezing back far enough to touch my spine. I hold this for the desired count and then repeat. Note: if you get light-headed at first and find it difficult to do four-second counts of box breathing, then start at two and a half or three seconds until this can be maintained, then gradually work your way up to four-second counts.

Box breathing is also great when you're starting to feel stressed or just prior to giving a presentation, speech, lesson, or sermon.

## INTERMEDIATE

# Breathe!
# (If You Wanna Live)

Exhale all of the air out of your lungs, then slowly breathe in a full breath at a four-second count, hold for four seconds, exhale for four seconds, and hold at the bottom for four seconds. Repeat for four cycles. An oxygenated mind is a mind that works more optimally.

**24**

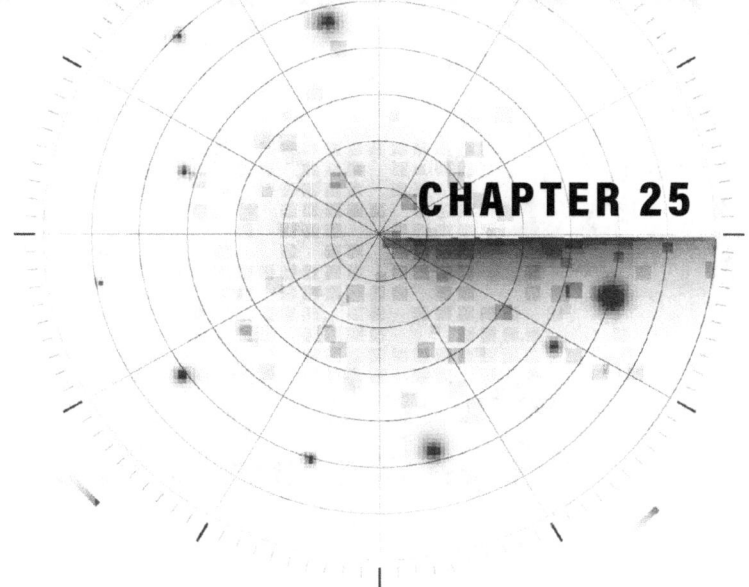

# CHAPTER 25

# OSWALD IS COMING

We all have our patterns. I'd be pretty easy to assassinate if someone knew my patterns. Would the same go for you? Do you take the same route to work every day, show up to the gym around the same time, park in the same area(s), stop at your favorite Starbucks?

### Exercise:

Find your patterns and write them out. Do you do things daily? Is there a Tuesday/Thursday or Monday/Wednesday/Friday pattern or pattern(s)? Change it up! Oswald is coming! Think back to Creature of Habit (chapter 2) and the lesson on creating alternate routes. Change your normal schedule for a week. Even if you have to take your kiddo to activities or classes on certain nights of the week, go a different route, show up earlier than normal, etc. The point is to not be so predictable. It's just one week, people! Git 'er done!

## INTERMEDIATE

## Oswald Is Coming

If you heard Lee Harvey Oswald was alive and was tracking you down, how easy would it be for him to do so? Practice alternating your routes, routines, and schedules (as much as possible) to not be so predictable.

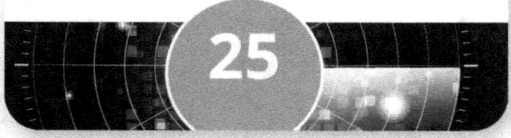

25

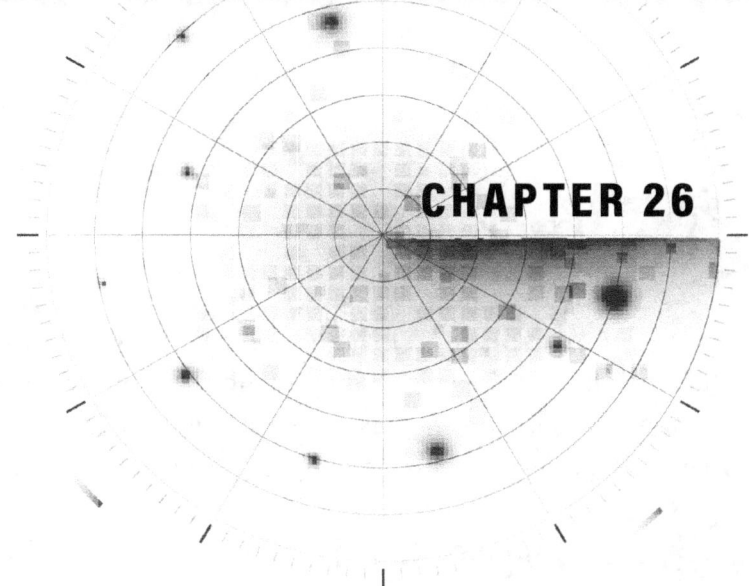

# CHAPTER 26

# GET SIDEWAYS

L ike in Chapter 27: Back It Up, Back It In, now you can begin. Try not to stand with your back facing anyone. Get sideways, and change position from time to time while keeping your head on a swivel (nonchalantly). I don't like crowds or standing in lines, like at TSA checkpoints at airports, because they herd you through a maze of cordoned-off pathways. There are generally no walls to back up to. It's very difficult to not have your back to someone at some point along the multiple twists and turns in line. Instead of just facing forward like a good boy, as all the other well-behaved children are doing, I stand sideways so I can use my peripheral vision and scan left to right. I face in the direction of what I assume are the most capable, sketchy people, and I'll adjust my sideways stance from time to time to Aim High (chapter 23) and soak in everything from far to near and near to far.

## Exercise:

For the next five days, expose as little of your front and back to people as possible. In law enforcement we call this "blading," which means standing with your gun/holster side away from anyone you might be confronting, asking questions of, or interviewing. This is a great practice for civilians to follow, as well.

## Things to Consider:

I'd rather be assaulted from directly in front of me versus from my back, but both our front and back sides have multiple areas of vulnerability which we should want to keep safe. Examples include the throat, eyes, groin, solar plexus, liver, and knees in the front; and the base of the skull, neck, spine, kidneys, hamstrings, and Achilles tendons in the back. Also, standing directly in front of or behind someone allows them the opportunity to attack you in a straight line across or perpendicular to the line your feet make (connecting the middle of each foot together with an invisible line), which could easily unbalance you and catch you flat-footed. This is why, when you watch folks playing tug-of-war, you see them pulling the rope as they keep their feet basically parallel to the direction of the rope they are pulling on. If one group stood with their feet parallel while the other group stood with their feet perpendicular to the pull rope, then the parallel-footed folks could be much weaker yet still prevail.

## Bonus:

Feeling is believing. I refer to the area where the middle of the feet connect with an invisible line as the *line of strength, power, and balance* (see Figures 1, 2, and 3). Stand facing a wall with your feet (foot line) parallel to the wall. You should be close enough to the wall that you could push off of it. Now, push off of the wall with some force and see how easy it is to displace your balance. Someone could also gently push you from behind, toward the wall, and you'd have to use your hands to catch your balance against the wall to avoid smacking into the wall in front of you. It's just as easy to pull someone backward from this position by grabbing their shoulders and pulling back perpendicular to the invisible line their feet make. You could also have someone push or pull you from the side, in line with your feet, and it becomes much harder (because you're stronger and more stable) for them to unbalance you, so long as the direction of force remains constant and in the same line.

**Figure 1**

# HEAD OVER BASE: POSTURE

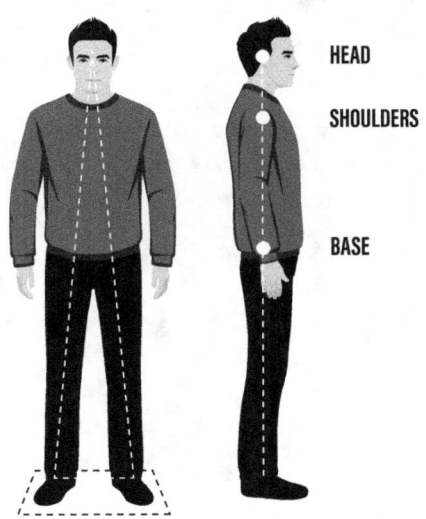

**Head Over Base:** Ears directly over shoulders; shoulders directly over hips.

To maintain balance, your head must be over your base (your base is your feet, or the box your feet would make if you drew a line around your toes, the outsides of your feet, and between your heels).

**Figure 2**

# LINE OF STRENGTH

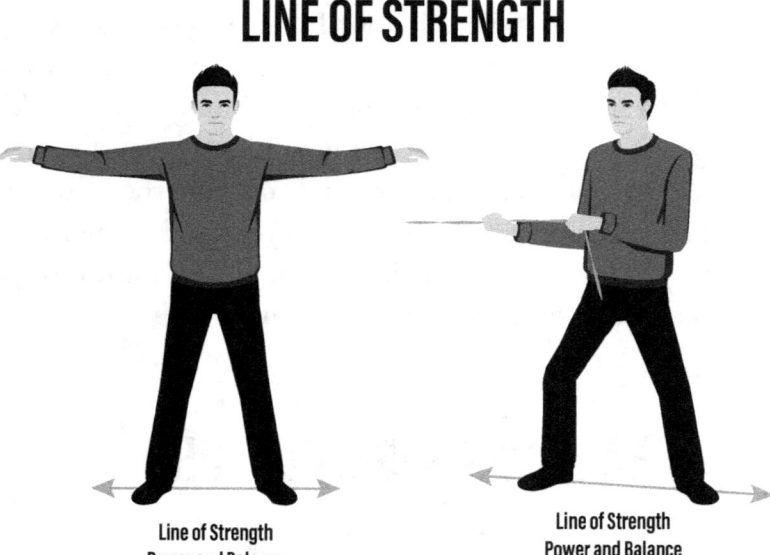

Line of Strength
Power and Balance

Line of Strength
Power and Balance

If you draw a line between the center of your feet, this is your line of strength, power, and balance. You're strong along this line, as demonstrated when maintaining a strong position in tug-of-war.

**Figure 3**

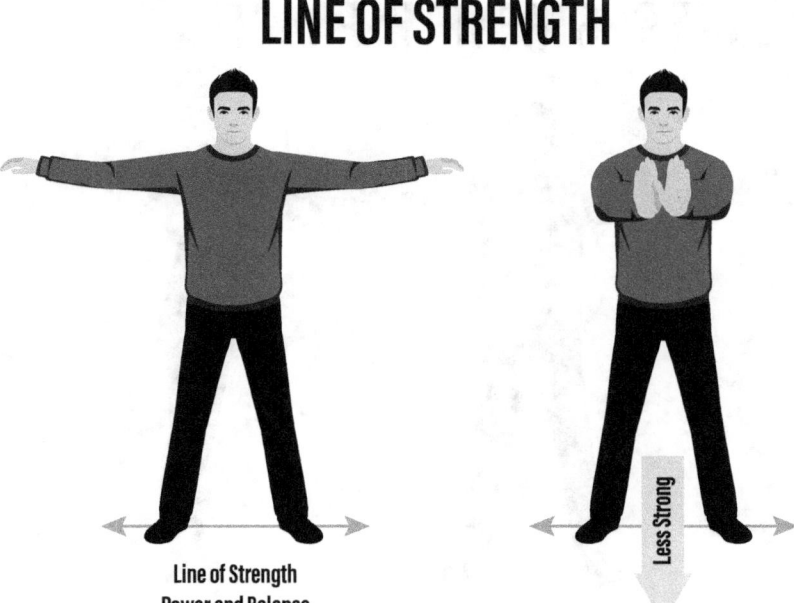

# LINE OF STRENGTH

**Line of Strength
Power and Balance**

The line perpendicular to your line of strength could be described as a line of weakness, or the line to use to unbalance someone. You could pull or push someone along this envisioned line to easily unbalance them, i.e., they would have to move their feet to try to reestablish their base; otherwise, they could easily fall if they keep their feet rooted in place.

**Figure 4**

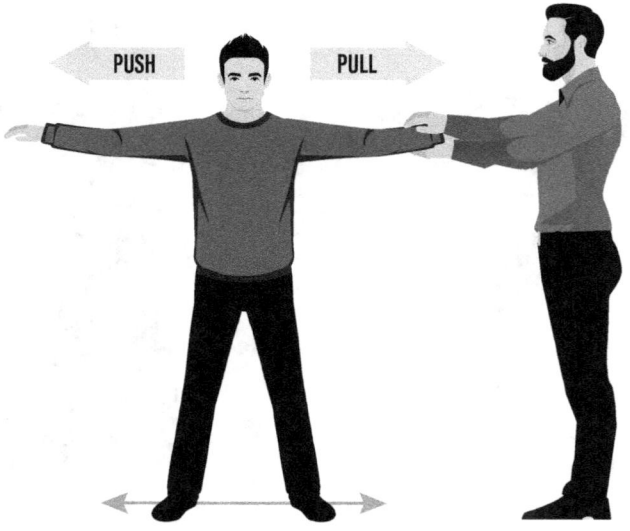

# LINE OF STRENGTH: PRACTICE 1

This image demonstrates that if I pull against someone along their line of strength, and they lean or resist in the opposite direction, they are in a strong position. The reverse is true: if I tried to push against them to unbalance them, and they leaned or resisted toward me, they again would be very strong along this line.

**Figure 5**

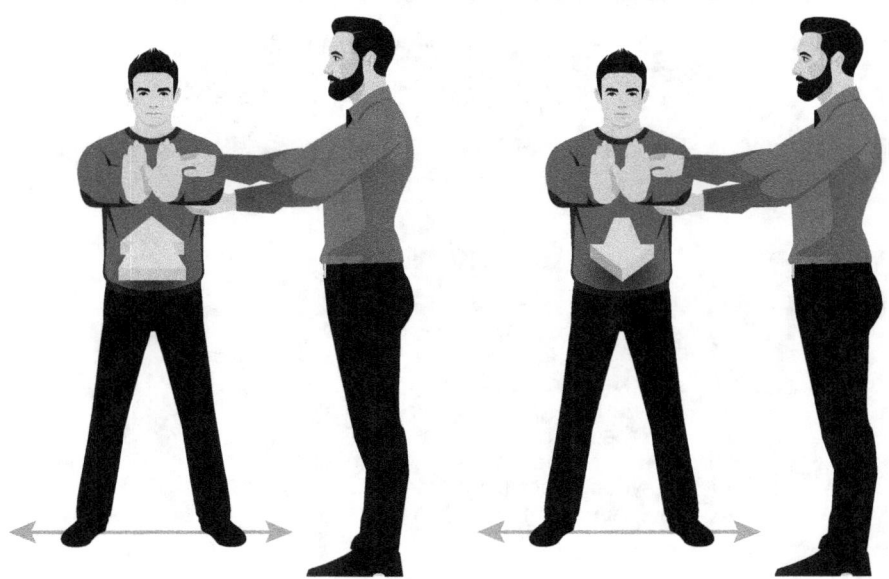

This image demonstrates pushing and pulling across the envisioned line of weakness, or the line to easily unbalance someone. If I pull or push them along this line, even if they resist, it is very easy for me to move their head beyond their base (or over, forward, or backward past their feet).

## INTERMEDIATE

### Get Sideways

Try not to stand with your back facing anyone. Get sideways and keep your head on a swivel. Use your peripheral vision and face in the direction of what you assume are the most sketchy people. Adjust your stance from time to time (23: Aim High) to soak in everything.

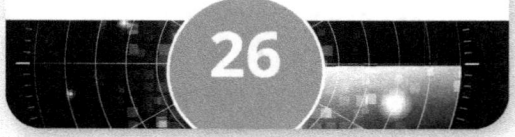

26

# ADVANCED

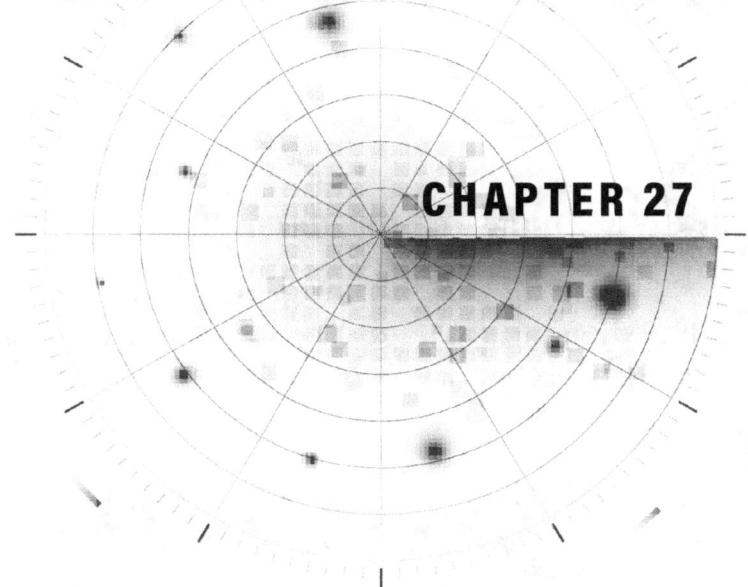

# CHAPTER 27

# BACK IT UP, BACK IT IN

N ow you can begin.

### Exercise:

Throughout the week, when you find yourself in a place where people are around you, don't expose your back to them. This is easier said than done. Whenever possible, put your back against a wall or a shelf in a grocery store aisle when you need to stop to read your shopping list or write a check (is that even a thing anymore?!). Do this for the next five days when in public.

## Things to Consider:

   If and when you can't put your back to a wall, column, shelf, etc., you might have to compromise. Feel free to revisit Chapter 26: Get Sideways and add it to this week's exercise.

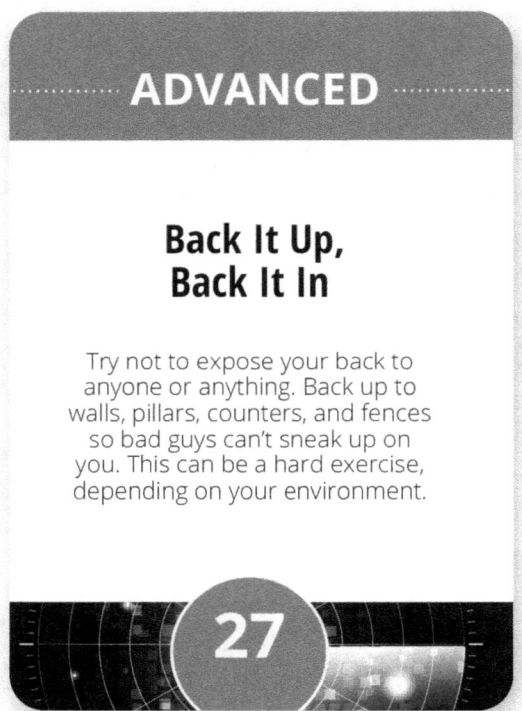

ADVANCED

### Back It Up, Back It In

Try not to expose your back to anyone or anything. Back up to walls, pillars, counters, and fences so bad guys can't sneak up on you. This can be a hard exercise, depending on your environment.

27

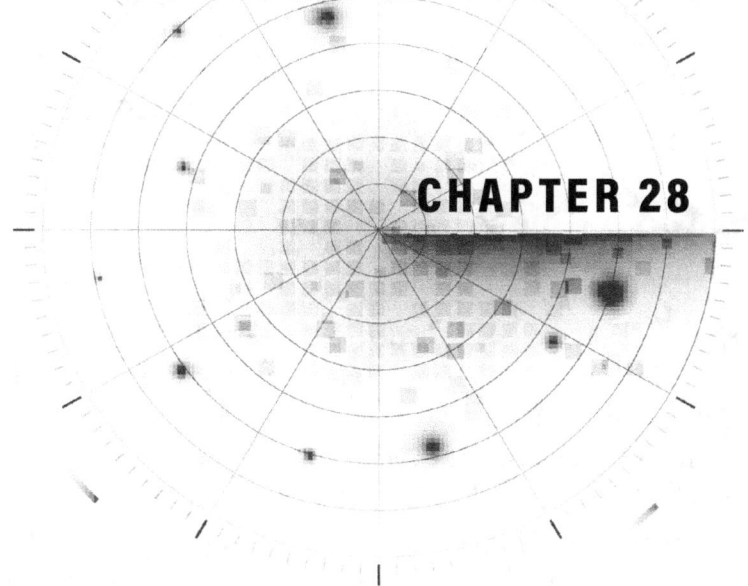

# CHAPTER 28

# VIBES

**T**his one is all about getting in touch with your feelings!

### Exercise:

Each day this week, wherever you find yourself in, tune in to any negative vibes you pick up on, not only the negative vibrations but also trying to pinpoint the source(s). Breathe, chill, get into a good mental space, and "tune in." If you're having trouble, revisit Chapter 24: *Breathe!* (If You Wanna Live) to assist you in this week's exercise and to help you open up and access the vibrations in your environment.

## Things to Consider:

When we think, we emit brain waves in a 360-degree spread. Women are particularly great at picking up on these signals. And, in the animal kingdom, dogs are the masters of tuning in. Before you open that door to scratch your dog behind the ears, they know, by feeling the vibes you're putting off, if you're in a good mood or a bad mood. I've had several doggies over the years (and still do), and when I get home, I'm either met by wagging tails or submissive whimpering based on the vibes I'm putting off. This is a great exercise to piggyback off of Chapter 8: Book by Its Cover. Vibes are a two-way street; you can also throw off vibes that say you aren't one to mess with, or vibes that are not aggressive or douchey (this could be a trigger for some) but confident. This is a great weekly exercise to hone when you're around someone who feels creepy and untrustworthy; if this is the case, treat them as such. We have instincts and a sixth sense for a reason. Thank you, good Lord, for this innate human ability, because it has literally saved my life on numerous occasions back when I was "Johnny Law" in Big D (Dallas, Texas).

We've all likely experienced and felt this. Have you ever been in a crowd when you got an uneasy feeling that you were being watched, only to turn your head in the direction you sensed it coming from and found someone from across the room staring at you? We all have this innate human ability, and not only that, but we can also pick up from a 360-degree field around our heads the general direction it's coming from. This is one reason I believe women are so good at it, because they get creeps looking at them and undressing them with their eyes all the time. Men, on the other hand, can get it often from a dude mean-muggin' the back of our head and visualizing doing bad things to us. Trust these instincts, and get good at tuning in to them. You can put off vibes—good or bad—that are laser-beam focused on one person. Just like the dude mean-muggin' the back of your head, you can do likewise to others, or you can send good "vibes" of positivity and healing intentions to people who seem to be having a crappy day. This is a kind of superpower (more on this later in this chapter).

As we'll touch on in Chapter 42: Walk the Walk, ditch the distractions in public. Walk with awareness, and remember what can happen in your brain. And skip ahead to the lesson from Chapter 43: Vision Quest: concentrating on a feed on your phone using focal vision will also hamper your ability to feel vibes. Also feel free to skip ahead to Chapter 36: Shock the Monkey to put that little primate in its place because it will also stuff your ability to be vibrationally aware.

And now for a personal share: As a police officer in Kerrville, Texas, I was getting called on the carpet and was being addressed by my superiors. There was one officer (a detective) in particular who I was at odds with. This was his choice, not mine. During the meeting, I was being asked a lot of questions regarding my judgment while I had been off duty in another city. Nothing bad at all had happened, but another officer from the Kerrville Police Department (KPD) had witnessed my antics at a bar while I was visiting some of my cop buddies from the Dallas Police Department. Yes, we can get a little crazy and fun-loving when we're out and about, especially in San Antonio. I knew the KPD superiors had nothing on me and were just fishing, trying to intimidate me and/or rattle my cage a bit. During the "talk," with a calm and innocent look on my face, while answering their questions, I was bombarding the detective (who didn't like me) with some "uncomfortable," highly focused vibes. Let's just say I was sending signals along with visualizations of what I'd "like" to do to him and how I'd physically carry them out, along with how easy it would be for me to accomplish these wishful musings. As it turned out, the detective kept squirming in his seat, he couldn't seem to get settled or comfortable, and the "interview" (which appeared at first to just be getting started) was abruptly called short and I was dismissed. I don't suggest you do this with folks you work with, especially if they have rank on you, because they will remember, and you'll have a target on your back. This guy disliked me even more after this incident. He eventually was in a position to get me kicked off the SWAT team by having the chief's ear, and he was one of the reasons I got out of law enforcement...I hated the big-city Dallas politics and the small-town Texas, good ole boy BS.

In contrast to the story above, there have been countless times when I've used vibes in good ways, to surround people with calming, soothing, peaceful, and healing vibes. This, when the other party is open to and can sense the vibes, is amazing to watch! You can almost see an instant change in their attitude, a deeper breath is taken, and a change in their body language comes over them. (Note to self: Do this more often! Spread some love!)

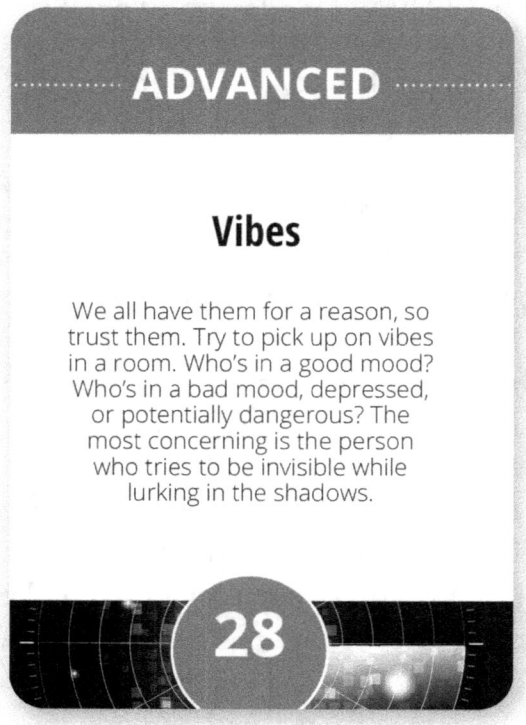

### ADVANCED

### Vibes

We all have them for a reason, so trust them. Try to pick up on vibes in a room. Who's in a good mood? Who's in a bad mood, depressed, or potentially dangerous? The most concerning is the person who tries to be invisible while lurking in the shadows.

28

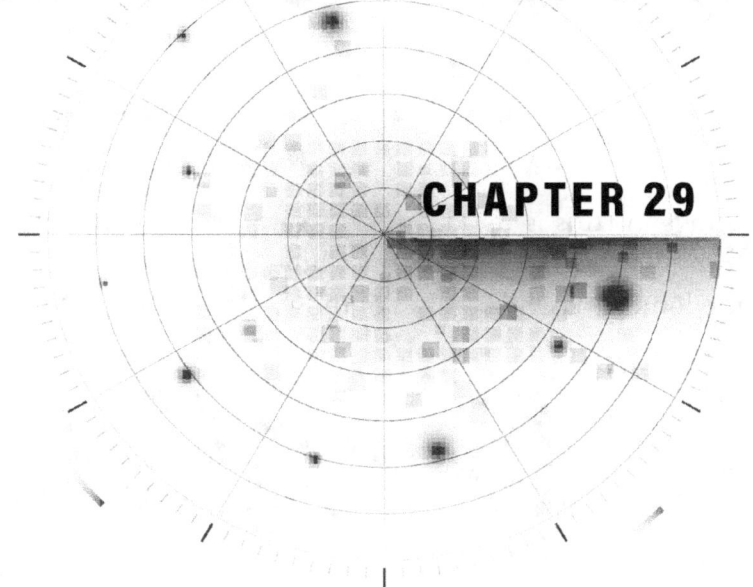

# CHAPTER 29

# WOLVES TRAVEL IN PACKS

L ook for the groups, but don't just look, *identify them*.

## Exercise:

Each day this week, look for and identify groups of people. Know their numbers, who the leader is, who the followers are, who wants to please the alpha, and who wants to replace the alpha. Are they a fair-weather band of frat bros whose bonds won't last after college? Or players in the sandbox who are brothers in arms? You better be able to discern the difference. Look for the wolves traveling in packs in food courts at the mall, at public gatherings, in stores, etc. Do they come together to talk and then spread out? Are they goofing around, up to trouble, or peeps just having fun? If there's a lookout who is holding back and taking things in (this is the dangerous coward), remember your exercises from Odd Man Out, Out for Chow, Weapons Inventory, and Case the Joint and piggyback off of those.

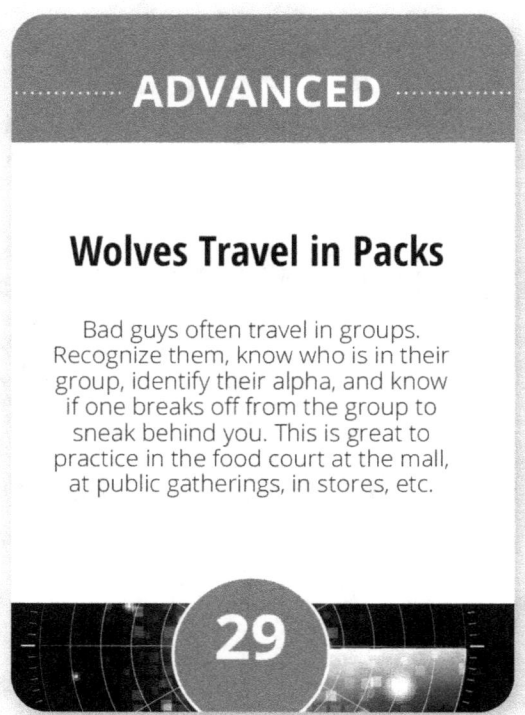

ADVANCED

## Wolves Travel in Packs

Bad guys often travel in groups. Recognize them, know who is in their group, identify their alpha, and know if one breaks off from the group to sneak behind you. This is great to practice in the food court at the mall, at public gatherings, in stores, etc.

29

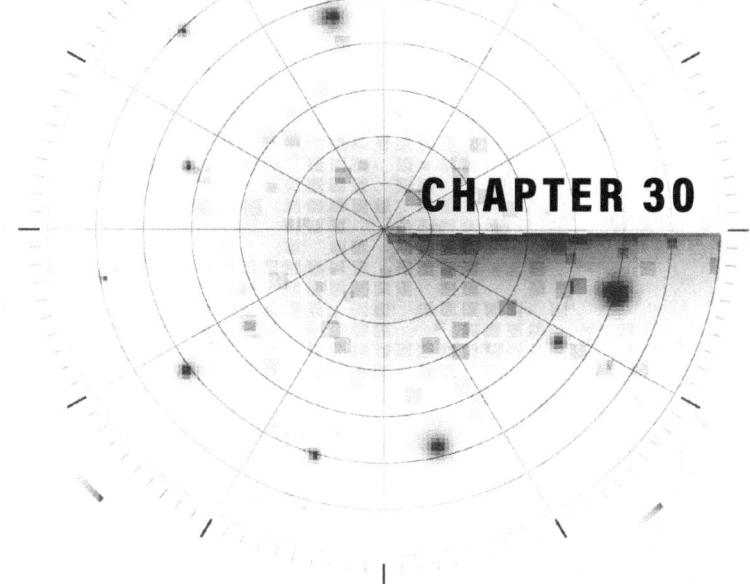

# CHAPTER 30

# KNOW YOUR FOREGROUND
# AND BACKGROUND

W̲e live in a three-dimensional world, and as such, we can be focused on one object or person and miss relevant details, objects, and people between and/or behind whatever has your attention.

## Exercise:

At least three times a day, for five days during the week, pick a target. If you had to make "the shot," what is between you and them? What is behind them if you miss or if the shot goes through them? You should also add to this week's exercise by reversing this. What if you were the target and the threat was coming from X direction? Where do you go? What do you do? Where is the closest cover? Do you have people you love and care about with you? How would you place yourself in relation to your loved ones? How many objects or barriers do you want between you and the threat from direction X? This also means getting off the X (which means getting off the point and place being targeted, which—in this scenario—is you).

## Things to Consider:

What are smart angles and straight lines to consider? And does it make sense to get low or move fast? FYI: a moving target is harder to hit!

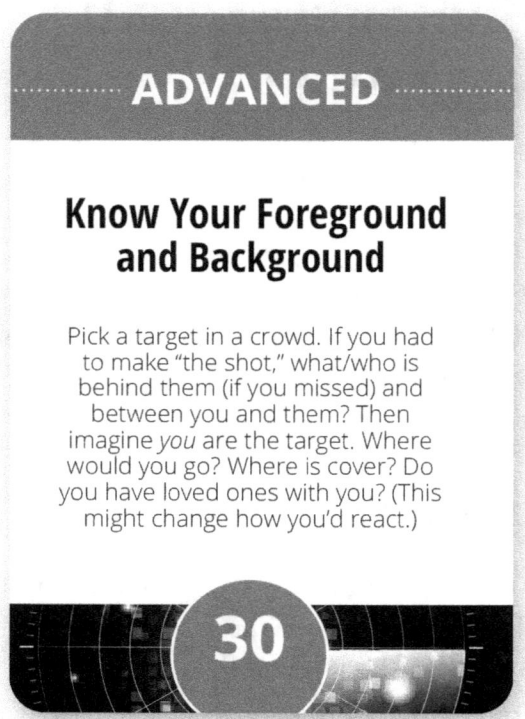

### ADVANCED

### Know Your Foreground and Background

Pick a target in a crowd. If you had to make "the shot," what/who is behind them (if you missed) and between you and them? Then imagine *you* are the target. Where would you go? Where is cover? Do you have loved ones with you? (This might change how you'd react.)

30

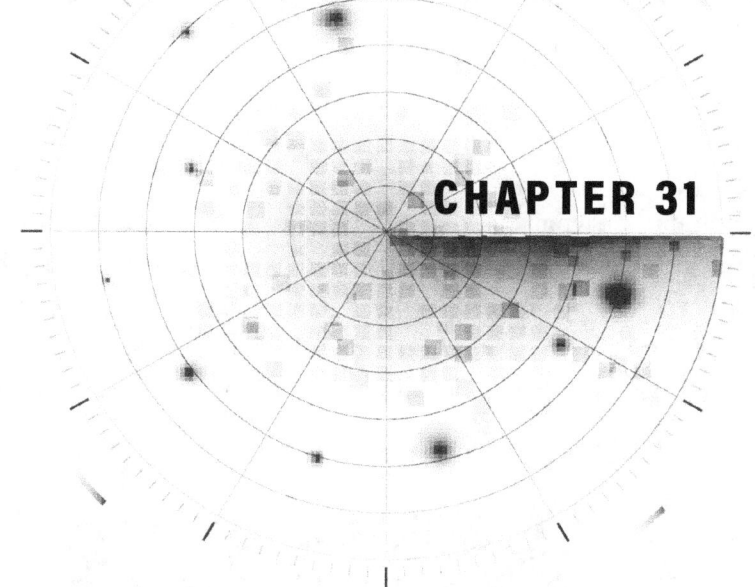

# CHAPTER 31

# GO DARK TO SEE THE LIGHT

**P**ower outages happen.

### Exercise:

Throughout the week, find all of the times when a flashlight would be useful, and in what situations or environmental conditions.

### Bonus:

Do your homework and read reviews on decent flashlights, including details like dependability, battery life, sturdiness, etc. Find out the size and number of lumens you think would be appropriate, and get used to having a flashlight on your person daily.

Remember what I said about it being better to have something and not need it than to need it and not have it? Portable flashlights are no exception. Oh, and I know many will say, "But my cell has one!" Get used to the phrase "two is one and one is none." Backups are essential because phones can break or go down, batteries die, etc.

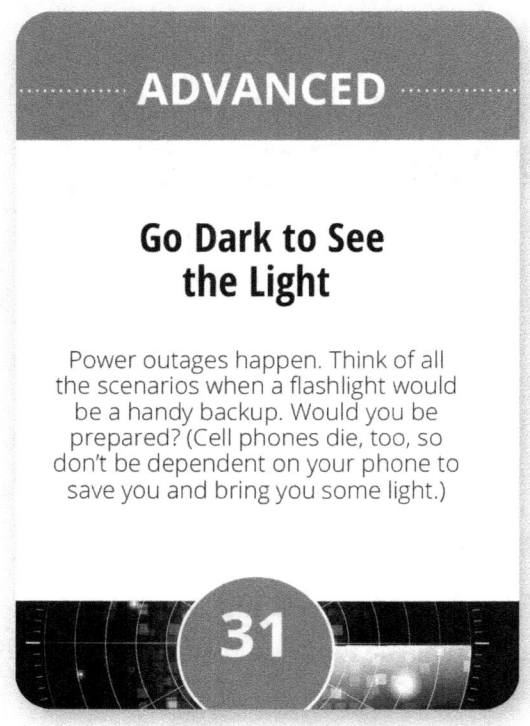

**ADVANCED**

## Go Dark to See the Light

Power outages happen. Think of all the scenarios when a flashlight would be a handy backup. Would you be prepared? (Cell phones die, too, so don't be dependent on your phone to save you and bring you some light.)

31

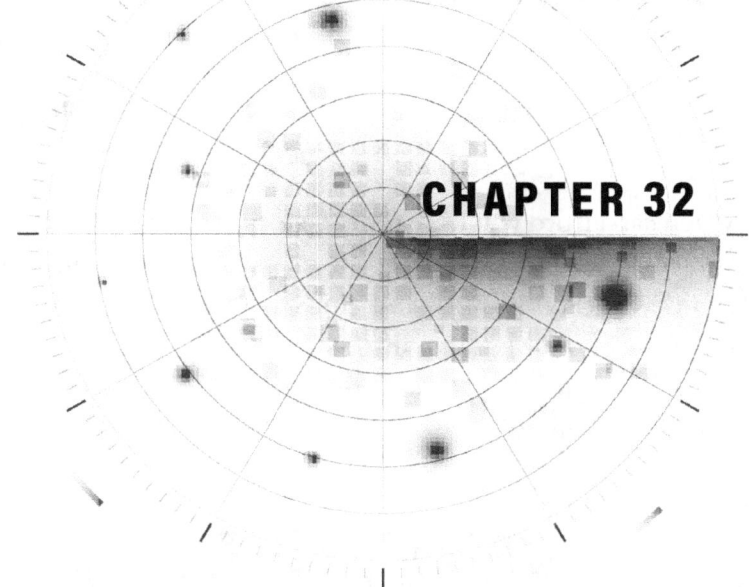

# CHAPTER 32

# OH MICKEY, YOU'RE SO FINE

**S**urround yourself with space when you're out and about and when in a vehicle.

### ⚙ Exercise:

Daily throughout the week, create a bubble of personal space around yourself and your vehicle. If something comes into your space, you'll have more time to react. I love this quote from Mickey Schuch, combative pistol instructor and founder of Carry Trainer: "Awareness is the currency with which you buy time to react." Truer words were never spoken. The only distance we can truly control in a vehicle is the space directly in front of us. Establish a four-second following distance when walking, jogging, biking, and driving. Travel in the "lane" of least resistance. This means surrounding yourself with space. Having space around you creates visibility, which can afford you time to react. Remember, a perfect-world strategy would be to create a bubble of space around you, which would afford you the visibility and time to react if something unwanted and/or undesirable came into your space. Don't get boxed in, leave yourself an out. If a person or a vehicle invades your bubble, you'll have more time to react.

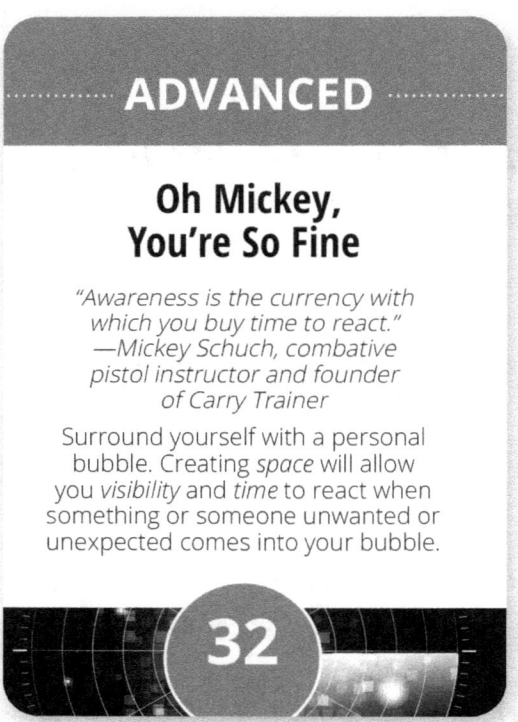

## ADVANCED

### Oh Mickey, You're So Fine

*"Awareness is the currency with which you buy time to react."*
*—Mickey Schuch, combative pistol instructor and founder of Carry Trainer*

Surround yourself with a personal bubble. Creating *space* will allow you *visibility* and *time* to react when something or someone unwanted or unexpected comes into your bubble.

32

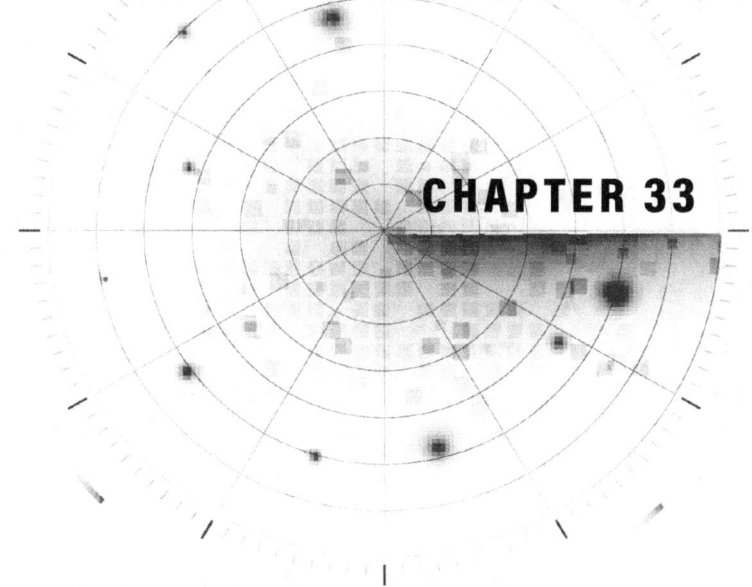

# CHAPTER 33

# LIGHT IT UP, UP, UP

H ow can you be aware in situations where there is poor lighting? Get a light! Now, you might be asking, "How do you make a weekly exercise out of this, Mr. Matt?" By coming up with different contingencies where having some light would/could be extremely useful and needed. Caveat: don't get super dependent upon them, because once the lights are up, you've just wrecked your night vision and that of those around you (and this works for the bad guys, too).

### Exercise:

"Light it up" in poor lighting situations, but *not* to the point where it totally blows your night vision. If you have a flashlight with a red or green filter over the lens, then awesome; otherwise, get good at cupping your hands over the lens and holding the flashlight behind you and off to one side of your body to give you the read of a room. You might not find yourself in poor lighting situations often, but if you go anywhere where there is electricity that can be turned off via a light switch, then make it a poor lighting situation and handle your business. This could be while cooking, showering, going to the restroom, getting dressed in the morning, etc. Each day this week, create a poor lighting situation and perform your task(s) while lighting it up...but not too much.

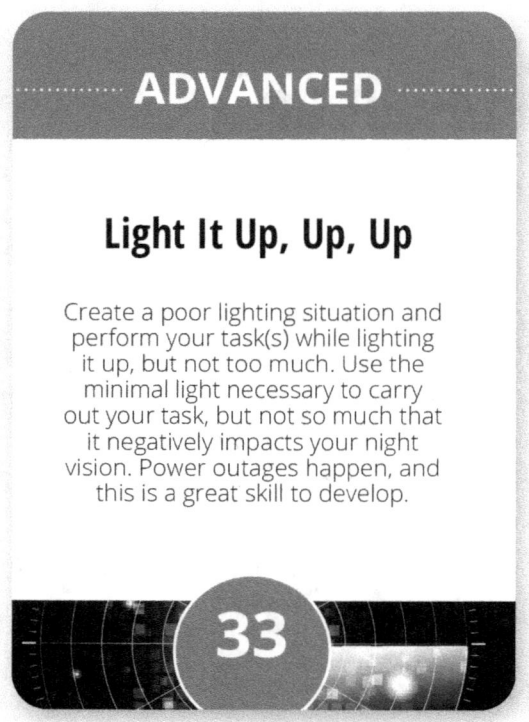

### ADVANCED

## Light It Up, Up, Up

Create a poor lighting situation and perform your task(s) while lighting it up, but not too much. Use the minimal light necessary to carry out your task, but not so much that it negatively impacts your night vision. Power outages happen, and this is a great skill to develop.

33

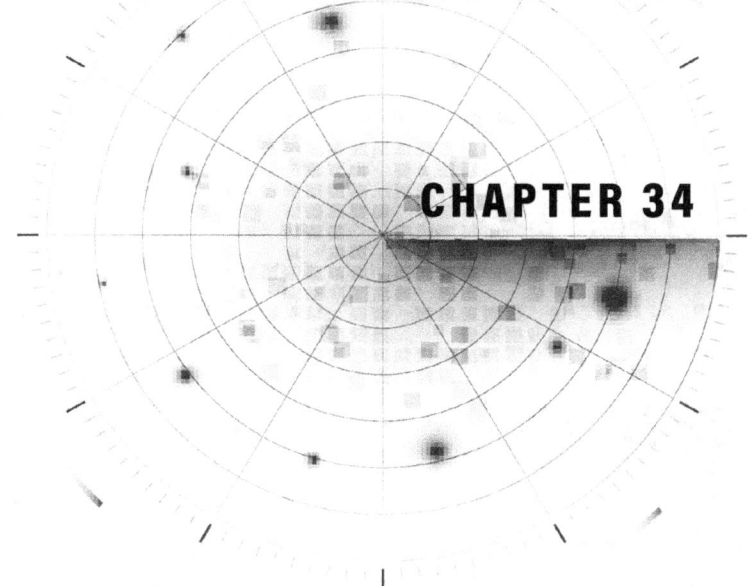

# AIN'T NO SUNSHINE

We have rods and cones in our eyes. We use rods for night vision and low light. There are over 100 million rod cells in the human eye, and only a few bits of light are needed to activate a rod. Unlike cones, rods don't help with color differentiation, which is why everything has a gray scale when we're using our night vision. This being said, we're at a disadvantage in low-light conditions because we can't optimally use all the benefits our eyes can offer in better lighting. Focal vision in low light can cause things to disappear. Unlike in Chapter 33: Light It Up, Up, Up, don't use another light source; just find low-light conditions, stare at something intently, and have it disappear by focusing on it. Look away and off of it, then back toward it, and you should be able to pick up what you're looking at again, especially if it's got movement. Our eyes are very good at picking up movement. Deer know this! They've been hunted for countless years. That's why they *freeze* when they feel threatened. Deer in the headlights...ring a bell? Deer also have adapted to feeding in low-light conditions as evolution has taught them that they have a better chance of survival when being hunted by human predators at times in the day when our eyes aren't working optimally.

## Exercise:

When there "ain't no sunshine" and you find yourself in a low-light situation (not so dark that you can't make things out), use focal vision and stare at something for several moments or minutes until it disappears. When it does, just like in Vision Quest (chapter 43), then bump your eyes left or right and up or down, and see the object or critter you were looking at come back into view. Do this ten to twenty times each evening or in low-light environments for the next five days.

## Bonus:

Don't just stare at something that's super close and easy to spot. Play with distances, shapes, and sizes of all objects, critters, and/or focal points to get a true feel for opening up your vision and being able to see what you want to see so you can sharpen your visual acuity and awareness. Also play with different levels of low light and/or changing light (ex: focus on dark shadows in your yard, and then focus across a lighted stretch of street into the next shadowed yard at your neighbor's distasteful, creepy yard gnome that's flippin' you the bird).

## ADVANCED

### Ain't No Sunshine

When you're in a low-light situation, use focal vision and stare at something for several moments until it disappears. When it does, bump your eyes left and right or up and down and see the object you were looking at come back into view. Do this ten to twenty times.

34

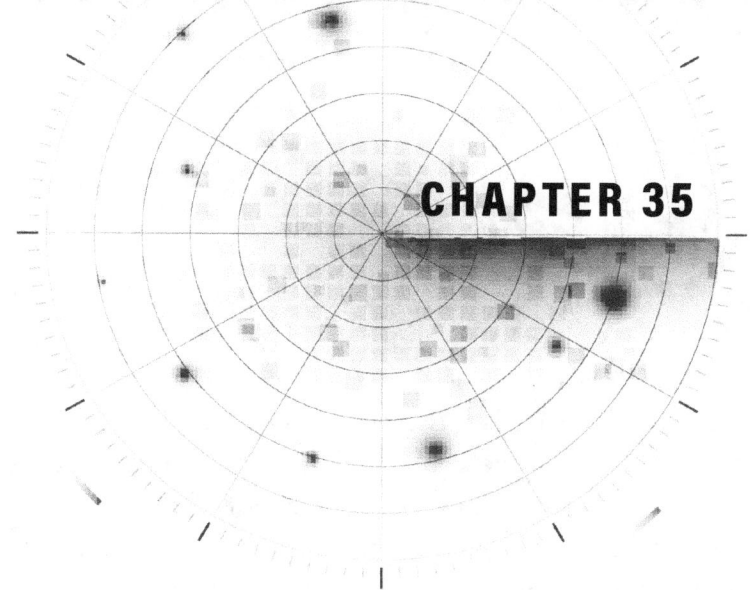

# CHAPTER 35

# MURPHY'S LAW

**W**hat can go wrong *will* go wrong, and at the most inopportune moment. Murphy's Law visualizations— these are an addition to the What-If Game (chapter 48). Visualize (with color and sound—screams and noises—make it as realistic as possible) that you are going through your scenarios with A, B, and C contingencies but things go wrong, less than perfect, or not how you (or those with you) would have optimally planned to react. See yourself dealing with snafus and succeeding anyway. Imagine tripping while running, going to a door to seek cover but the door happens to be locked, etc. The important thing here is to visualize—see and feel yourself—running through these mental scenarios and winning, living to fight another day. Make sure you always win, even though perhaps you'll be a bit battered and bruised with skinned knees. And *always* anchor and end the visualization exercise with positive thoughts. Feel the elation and emotion of being a badass survivor!

# Exercise:

During the week, pick places and times to "what if, but then." Let's piggyback off of the what-if scenarios from Chapter 48: The What-If Game. The point of this week's exercise is to bake in go-to actions based on the what-if scenarios you've created; only this time, things don't go as planned. It is likely things won't go perfectly, which is Murphy's Law, so visualize less-than-optimal hiccups and conflicts as you work through your mental contingencies *but* succeed and survive, regardless of added complications and inconveniences.

If you find it challenging to come up with weekly snafus to have to deal with, I've added some thoughts and examples below.

**Day 1—At a Restaurant:** A man walks in the front door and starts shooting randomly in all different directions. Where do you go, and what do you do?
*With Murphy the Mofo:* You have family with you, and you've twisted, sprained, or strained your knee or ankle, and one leg can't bear your full weight. Where do you go, and what do you do?

**Day 2—At work:** You're in your office or cubicle, typing away, and you hear gunshots from another side of the building, but you can't see the gunman. Where do you go, and what do you do? If you work from home, get creative. Imagine you hear sirens getting louder and coming toward your street, or you hear a car crashing into some vehicles parked along your street. Or you see two guys jumping out of a car, one flees across the street and the other heads toward your house and jumps the fence into your backyard as police squad cars come screeching to a stop in front of your place. Where do you go, and what do you do? And here's a little nuance to the above, if you're in an apartment, duplex, etc. Imagine the same scenario as above, but the one suspect runs toward your building, floor, etc. and soon afterward, the squad cars pull up and you hear someone on the other side of your door trying to open it. Where do you go, and what do you do?

*With Murphy the Mofo:* The fleeing suspect kicks in your door and makes entry! Where do you go, and what do you do?

**Day 3—In Public:** You're in a restroom and you hear a massive explosion not far off that rocks the building, shaking it and shuddering it. The power goes out. Where do you go, and what do you do?

*With Murphy the Mofo:* Your cell phone just died, and you don't have a flashlight (or the battery is dead...they do that, you know)! Where do you go, and what do you do?

**Day 4—While Driving:** You're passing an eighteen-wheeler semitrailer (or it's passing you) when one of its outside tires blow. The rubber shreds sling off of the rim and slap the front of your windshield. Where do you go, and what do you do?

*With Murphy the Mofo:* The impact to your windshield deploys your vehicle's airbags. Your hands snap off the wheel and that BS powder from the deployed airbag fills your vehicle's interior, making it hard to see and quickly creating a breathing irritant. Where do you go, and what do you do?

**Day 5—Road Rage:** Someone is riding your bumper, and as they pass you with all their impatience, they honk, flip you the bird, and pull in front of you. They then start and stop, braking hard in front of you and forcing you to brake to avoid rear-ending them. Where do you go, and what do you do?

*With Murphy the Mofo:* The jerk stops brake-checking you and pulls off into a parking lot, only to get behind you again after you've passed them. You're not alone, you have one or more loved ones in the car with you. The other driver starts riding your bumper uncomfortably close. Where do you go, and what do you do?

## ADVANCED

# Murphy's Law

It is likely things won't go perfectly, which is Murphy's Law. Piggybacking off of your scenarios from 48: The What-If Game, visualize less-than-optimal hiccups and conflicts as you work through your mental contingencies *but* succeed and survive regardless of added complications and inconveniences.

**35**

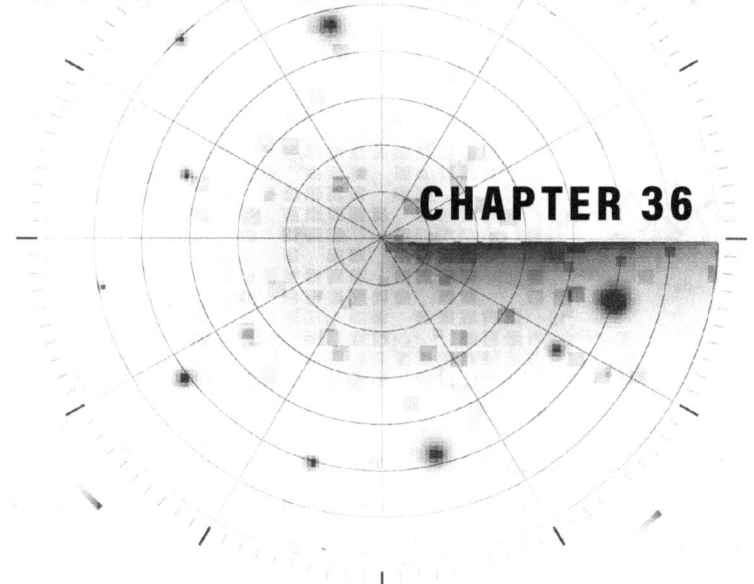

# CHAPTER 36

# SHOCK THE MONKEY

**B**e in the present moment. Don't let background mind chatter get in the way of being fully present to focus on the cognitive skills needed to accomplish what you're trying to accomplish.

## Exercise:

Five times a day, set a timer for five minutes and allow yourself to be totally immersed in taking in all of the environmental information around you, or to focus completely on the task you're working on. It's not as easy as it sounds. Your mind will drift to honey-dos, laundry lists, etc., but it's super important to be able to recognize this scatterbrained, hyper, needy "monkey" that lives in the back of your mind, screaming incessantly at all the things you *must* do and jumping from one subject to another like a spaz. Eastern philosophies such as Buddhism, Zen, Taoism, and neo-Confucianism call this the *monkey mind* or *mind monkey*.

## Things to Consider:

I'm taking liberties in my translation and explanation, and I'm honing in on a narrow part of the monkey mind, i.e., the conscious part of you that can be very distracting. Know that being in a conscious state isn't always bad when it comes to being situationally aware; in fact, it's needed quite often. But here I'm specifically calling out the rascal of an annoying monkey that's screaming in the back of your head, negatively affecting your clear decision-making. You have likely experienced this before. Have you ever driven down a highway or interstate with your eyes wide open and looking straight ahead, seemingly "aware," when you realize you've just passed your exit? You were mentally distracted, paying bills in your head, zonin' out. Shock the heck outta that dang monkey and put him in time-out! You have to ignore the monkey mind and truly live in the present moment, second by second, to be fully situationally aware. After all, your life and the lives of those you love may very well depend on it. After you've consistently hit your five-minute goal, expand upon your times performed per day as well as the duration of minutes spent. This isn't brows-furrowed, vein-popping-out-of-your-head concentration. Relax, chill, soak it all in, be the observer. Use as many of your senses as you can. Take in all the sights, sounds, temperature, and air flow, and just *be* in an aware state.

## ADVANCED

# Shock the Monkey

Five times a day, set a timer for five
minutes to be totally immersed
in the environmental information
around you or to focus completely
on the task you're working on. As
time goes on, increase the time
you spend being immersed and
focused on environmental inputs
and/or your chosen task(s).

36

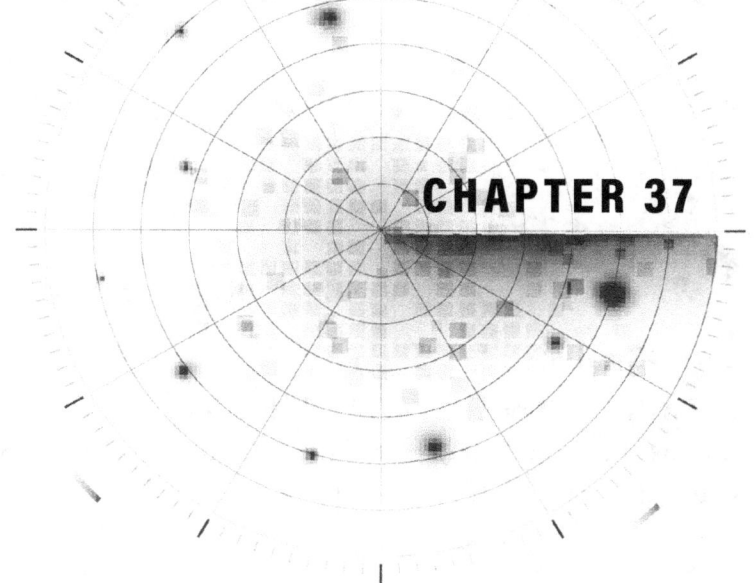

# CHAPTER 37

# WITH BLINDERS ON

ike in Shock the Monkey (chapter 36), be in the present moment. Do this in a safe place; don't do this while you're driving or when sitting at a crowded bus stop with hoods (bad characters) around.

## Exercise:

Take away your sense of sight and pay attention to noises and sounds around you. Intermittently pick a sound, noise, or movement to pay particular attention to. Mentally judge how far (distance and direction, if applicable) that noise/sound/movement is from you, and then open your eyes to validate. Like when practicing Shock the Monkey, set a timer for five minutes, and do this five times a day to be totally immersed in taking in all the environmental information around you. Up your time and duration based on your success and ability to truly concentrate.

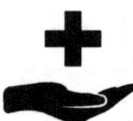

## Bonus:

Get really good at this with noises behind you.

### Extra Bonus:

Do this while performing Shock the Monkey, but key in on noises, sounds, etc. from behind you, and then turn your head to validate if you had identified them correctly.

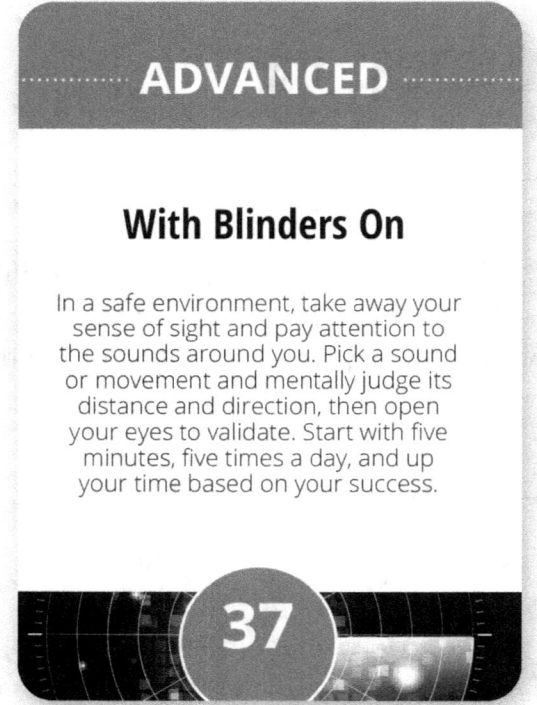

**ADVANCED**

## With Blinders On

In a safe environment, take away your sense of sight and pay attention to the sounds around you. Pick a sound or movement and mentally judge its distance and direction, then open your eyes to validate. Start with five minutes, five times a day, and up your time based on your success.

37

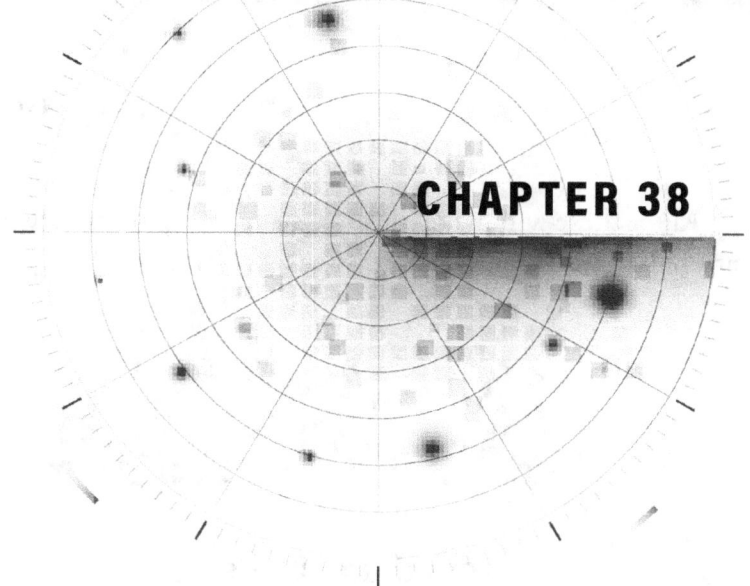

# CHAPTER 38

# LESS THAN 100 PERCENT

**T**his exercise is to be used in conjunction with the chapters that have already been drilled.

## Exercise:

Pick one, two, or three previous weekly exercises (and/ or incorporate several together), and do them at less than 100 percent. For example:

- Day 1: Only use one eye.
- Day 2: Use earplugs (to mimic impaired hearing).
- Day 3: Skip a meal or two (to simulate being very hungry).
- Day 4: Don't use your dominant arm or hand.
- Day 5: Get a few less hours of sleep than usual (as though you were sleep-deprived).

All of these will make it more challenging to concentrate on situational awareness and can cause easy frustration(s).

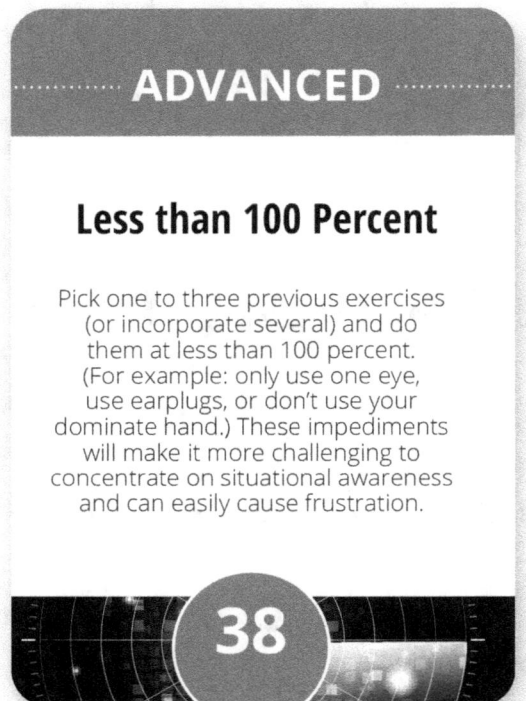

## ADVANCED

### Less than 100 Percent

Pick one to three previous exercises (or incorporate several) and do them at less than 100 percent. (For example: only use one eye, use earplugs, or don't use your dominate hand.) These impediments will make it more challenging to concentrate on situational awareness and can easily cause frustration.

**38**

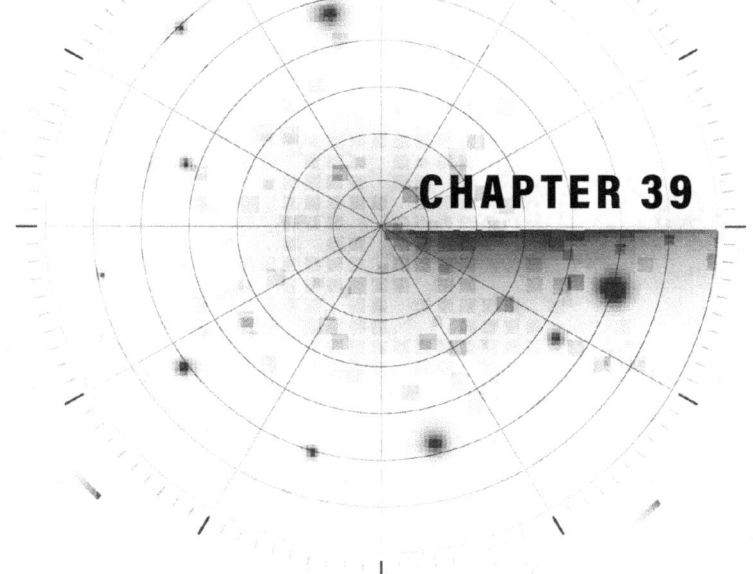

# CHAPTER 39

# BODYGUARD

Being situationally aware for your own safety is one thing, but the reality is, you also have loved ones in your life, and you'll want to care for their safety and well-being as much (if not more than) your own.

### Exercise:

Be situationally aware for someone else. This is easy to pull off with your spouse and/or children.

### Bonus:

Do the same for a stranger (it can be from afar) without them knowing. (To avoid getting caught and labeled as a creep!)

## Things to Consider:

This one for me is a constant, and it's likely one of the most practiced situational awareness drills I use each and every time I'm out with my wife and/or my daughter. There are several reasons for this:

1. It is *my job* as a husband/spouse and father/parent to live this way.

   A. It's also my job to do it in a subtle way so that they feel comfortable being themselves when I happen to be out with them in public. There's nothing worse than a killjoy dad with a scowl on his face who's mean-muggin' everyone he crosses paths with. There are, however, times when my radar gets set off and I'm visibly uncomfortable. In these moments, my wife and daughter can feel it, and they know something is up with me. Usually, at times like this, I just suggest we wrap up whatever we're doing and move venues, go to the next store, whatever, which solves the situation 99.9 percent of the time. Often it can be a crowd that sets off my alarm bells. The sheer number of people for me to keep tabs on creates a stressful and high-pressure situation because I can't watch everyone at once or to the level of attention I'd prefer. Using many of the techniques in this book allows for great success, even when I'm solo, and especially when I'm getting vibes from certain areas, groups, and pockets of people in crowded venues and spaces.

   B. Note: If you have a partner who also knows these exercises, you can split the space and agree on sectors to keep tabs on, which makes this much more doable. You have to be able to trust this partner and their ability to be a good bodyguard for their area of responsibility; otherwise, you're back in the first scenario where you have to do your work and double-check theirs. The bonus payoff for someone who is capable as a partner is that you also immediately have backup if a SHTF scenario goes down.

    i. If you partner up with one or more people in this exercise, don't forget the A, B, and C contingencies and the priorities of action. For example, if a bang goes off in the area, I'll grab the rest of our group and we'll leapfrog to exit A; if that's not viable, we'll immediately go to exit B. My partner knows to leapfrog behind us and will remain focused on the area of threat, ready, willing, and able to lay down withering cover fire should the bad guys choose to pursue, or if the situation calls for it.

C. Another note: Having trusted partners is great, especially if you've been in high-pressure situations in the past, because you've established trust and can move in sync without having to speak, you just act. However, even if you have superhero powers and situational awareness comes as easily to you as brushing your teeth, preplanning and having a premortem are always best practices. Remember Murphy's Law (chapter 35), stay positive, and *win*. This is about using your wisdom versus assuming we all have the same plan for getting off the X when the SHTF.

2. Most people are horribly situationally aware. And even if some are *somewhat* and *sometimes* aware, they can miss key details, people, hints, cues, and clues that a good bodyguard won't.

3. I don't necessarily want the person or people I'm with to *not* have a great, enjoyable time while we're out. I can bodyguard and leave them to focal-vision on price tags at the thrift store while I do what comes naturally to me based on my nature, training, and the nonnegotiable tenets I stand for.

Sometimes we're out with more folks, such as on a family outing with extended family, friends, and loved ones. This adds more elements to the mix, more situationally unaware folks, and more practice for me.

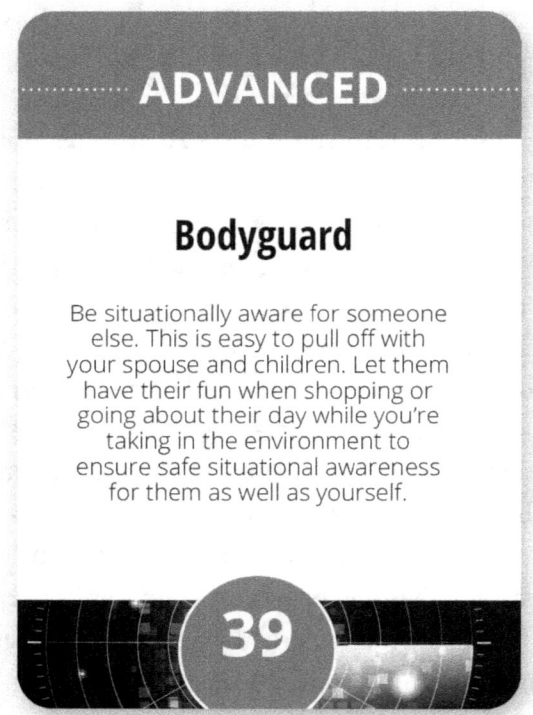

## ADVANCED

### Bodyguard

Be situationally aware for someone else. This is easy to pull off with your spouse and children. Let them have their fun when shopping or going about their day while you're taking in the environment to ensure safe situational awareness for them as well as yourself.

**39**

# TOP TIER

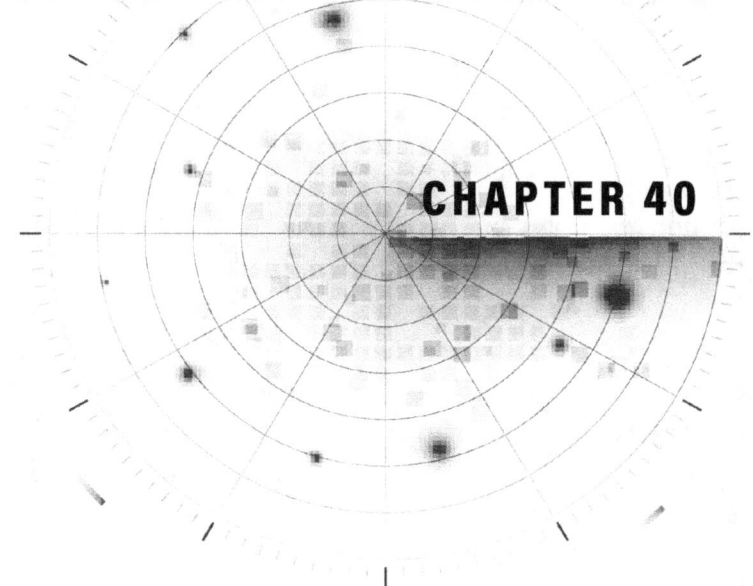

# CHAPTER 40

# CONCEALMENT VERSUS COVER

Inside or outside, know what concealment is and know what cover is. Think of concealment as a bedsheet or a shower curtain; you can't see me, but the bedsheet or curtain is easily penetrable by bad things that can hurt me. Cover is anything that can stop, impede, or deflect incoming rounds (like a brick wall). Cover can bonus as concealment (like a thick-trunked, mighty oak), or it can just be cover (such as bulletproof glass). The purpose of identifying this on the daily is to embed go-tos in your subconscious so that when the SHTF, you don't have to think, you'll just *go*—hopefully. You must exercise this drill with a priority focus, first on cover and secondarily on concealment. Concealment isn't "bad," depending on the circumstances, and it's better than nothing. If a bad guy can't see where I am to shoot at me, that's good for me and bad for him.

When you're identifying areas for concealment and cover, keep in mind that your home and office walls and cubicles are all concealment at best (in most cases). This is because, depending on the rounds a shooter might be using, there are several that will blow through drywall like a hot knife through butter. Know this and take in your environment accordingly.

Regarding outside environments (parking lots and such), vehicles can often provide decent cover, but know where to hide behind a vehicle. The damn movies often show cops squatting behind an open squad car door for cover while shooting pistols at bad guys toting AK-47s. This is movie fluff, so don't base your tactics on Hollywood bull dookie. Doors and glass are concealment at best, and if you're hiding in a vehicle (no matter the size), your movement is limited. Also, vehicles rock and move when people jostle around inside. Remember: eyes are attracted to movement, even subtle or slight movements, and even at a distance (more on the eyes in Chapter 43: Vision Quest). This is an innate human gift that was passed down from our ancestors when they were hunted by big-ass dinosaurs and saber-toothed tigers. Ask yourself: front or backside of a vehicle, when hiding? If it's diesel, propane, or gas-powered, stay away from those fuel tanks! Traditional gas guzzlers have tanks in the back and engine blocks in the front. Pick the engine block end of the ride. Also think about the axles. If I was a bad guy, and I saw feet or a squatting body (cast by a shadow—yup, the sun and shadows can give you away) hiding on the other side of a vehicle, and I wanted a higher head count, I'd drop to a knee and start walking rounds from my side of the car to the side where they are hiding to ric (ricochet) BBs off the pavement to chew them up. Hide behind an axle, preferably the front axle, behind the engine block (if the gas tank is in the rear).

## Exercise:

To put this into practice, identify all points, places, and things that are cover and concealment. Do this every day for a week for each place you visit. In a perfect world, cover is best because it can offer concealment with the added bonus of being cover. But concealment shouldn't be automatically overlooked and discounted. If I can't be seen, to be made an easy target of, then good for me and bad for the bad guy.

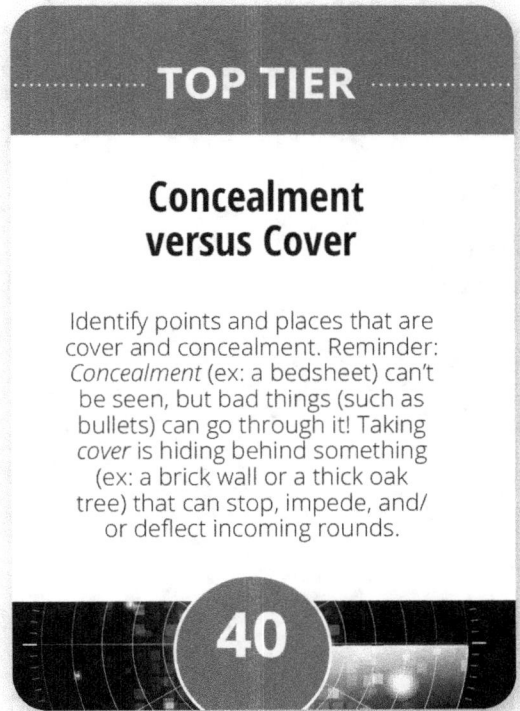

## Things to Consider:

What are you wearing? Unless you leave the house in camo that is perfectly suited for the office building's shrubbery you're attempting to hide behind, you'll likely not be hidden. Seasons matter when it comes to hiding behind foliage; spring, summer, winter, and fall will vary in the degrees of concealment they provide as well as what clothing could or couldn't assist you in being concealed. If you're hiding, be still and get low. Remember what was said earlier about the eyes and their attraction to movement.

### TOP TIER

### Concealment versus Cover

Identify points and places that are cover and concealment. Reminder: *Concealment* (ex: a bedsheet) can't be seen, but bad things (such as bullets) can go through it! Taking *cover* is hiding behind something (ex: a brick wall or a thick oak tree) that can stop, impede, and/ or deflect incoming rounds.

**40**

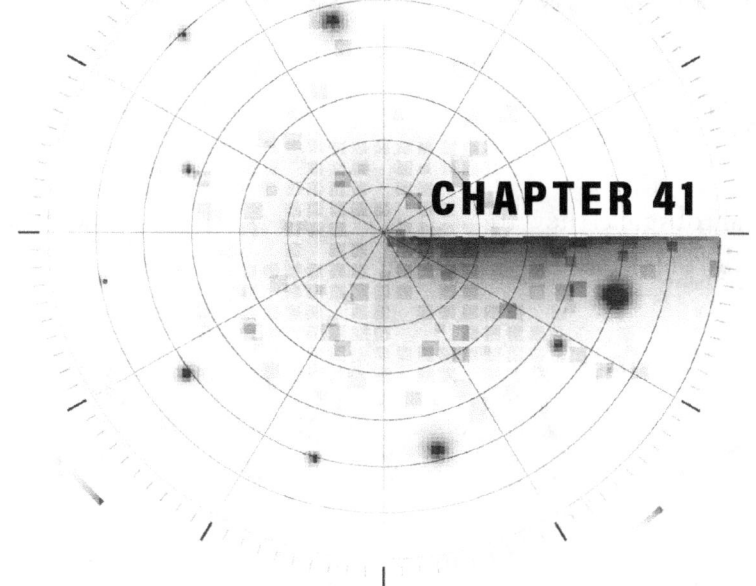

# CHAPTER 41

# TAG, YOU'RE IT

Proximity awareness training: How many people could you walk up to, touch, and say, "Tag, you're it"? How many people could do it to you?

### Exercise:

During this week's exercise, get close enough to tag unaware folks (but don't actually do it, unless you want trouble). And don't let anyone who isn't a family member, friend, or acquaintance get close enough to tag you. If they can touch you, they can hurt you. Play solo, if possible, in every place you visit over the next five days. You'll be amazed at how many folks lack situational awareness and are walking through life clueless, and you might be surprised by those who do have that awareness. You might also be surprised by those who get closer to you than you want them to when they *aren't* necessarily meaning to, they're just going about their day and you're an obstacle they are trying to get around—and they aren't playing the tag game like you are.

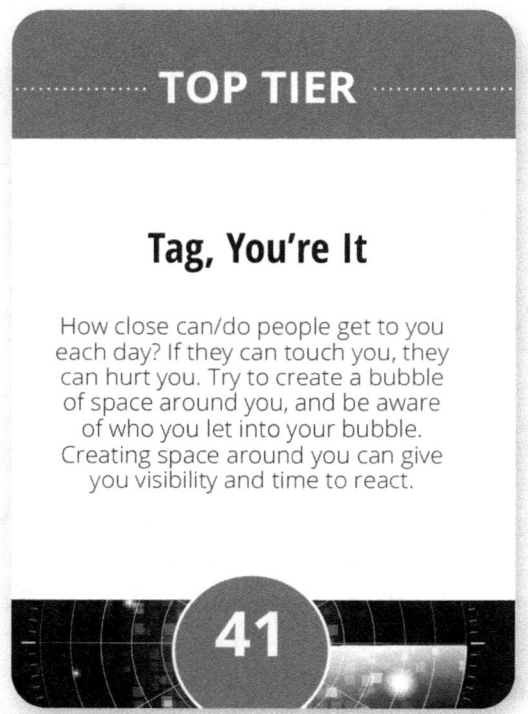

TOP TIER

## Tag, You're It

How close can/do people get to you each day? If they can touch you, they can hurt you. Try to create a bubble of space around you, and be aware of who you let into your bubble. Creating space around you can give you visibility and time to react.

41

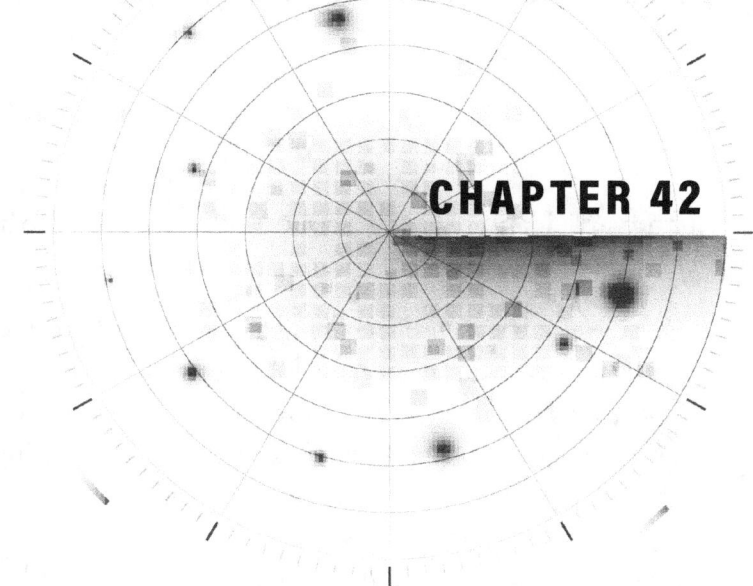

# CHAPTER 42

# WALK THE WALK

**W**alk with your back straight and aim to appear confident, with your head on a swivel, always aware of your surroundings. Ditch the distractions in public. Walk with awareness and look confident, versus looking like easy *prey* for the predator(s). There is a time and place to use your cell phone. Just like you would ditch the cell phone and other distractions when you're driving, the same is true for when you're walking, pedestrian-style, as you interact with your environment.

There's some science behind this, and you need to understand what you are giving up by choosing to multitask. The Carnegie Mellon University Study[1] took fMRIs (functional magnetic resonance imaging) of participants' brains while they used driving simulators. The researchers then compared those images against images recorded

---

1    Marcel Adam Just, Timothy A. Keller, and Jacquelyn Cynkar, "A Decrease in Brain Activation Associated with Driving When Listening to Someone Speak," *Brain Research* 1205 (2008): 70–80, https://doi.org/10.1016/j.brainres.2007.12.075.

when the participants drove the same simulators while also listening to sentences being read over headphones. Here are some of their findings:

- Just listening to sentences being read over headphones decreased activity in the brain's parietal lobe by 37 percent. This is the area of the brain that perceives movement, integrates sensory information, and is also important for language processing.
- Listening and language comprehension drew cognitive resources away from driving.
- It also decreased activity in the brain's occipital lobe, which processes visual information.

The takeaways: From this study, we can see that multitasking in this way takes 37 percent of the cognitive skills and brain functions away from the act of paying full attention to our current activity which, in this case, was operating a driving simulator (see Figure 1). So, if you're driving while talking on a cell phone, the best grade you can get—even if you're talking hands-free—is a D:

100% – 37% = 63%

**Figure 1**

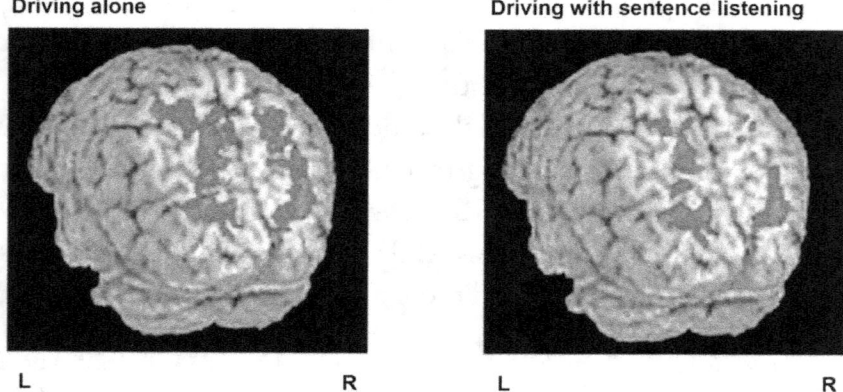

Functional magnetic resonance imaging images.
Source: Carnegie Mellon University

I don't know about you, but my ma wouldn't have been jazzed if I came home and bragged about getting a 63 on a final exam. If you see a distracted driver on the road near you, passing you, or tailgating you, then understand that they are a D at best. Feel free to make the D stand for something...I do! (Dummy, Dunce, Douchebag, etc.) Then get the heck away from them.

This multitasking brain drain also happens when we're not driving. As noted in the study, comprehension drew cognitive resources away from awareness, and it also decreased activity in the area of the brain that's responsible for processing visual information. We'll talk more about vision in Chapter 43: Vision Quest.

## ⚙️ Exercise:

When I say to keep your head on a swivel, I don't mean a crazy, paranoid, stare-people-down, psycho look (this could trigger some predators and can make you stand out). So, drop the crazy, but be aware, telling the world you're not an easy target. Make brief eye contact, and if you see someone looking at you, give them a slight head nod with your brows lowered in a look of semi- concentration (not an angry face or a frown, but as if you're thinking of your shopping list). The brief eye contact lets them know you have seen them, without having a stare-down contest that could elicit any aggression. You can also use the open vision we'll talk about in Chapter 43: Vision Quest, and other tactics covered in Chapter 47: Mirror, Mirror on the Wall, to be aware of their location without looking directly at them.

## TOP TIER

# Walk the Walk

Walk with confidence. Stand straight and keep your head on a swivel; be aware of your surroundings. Make brief eye contact with others, and if you see someone looking at you, give them a slight nod so they'll know you've seen them. Don't look like a potential victim to predators.

**42**

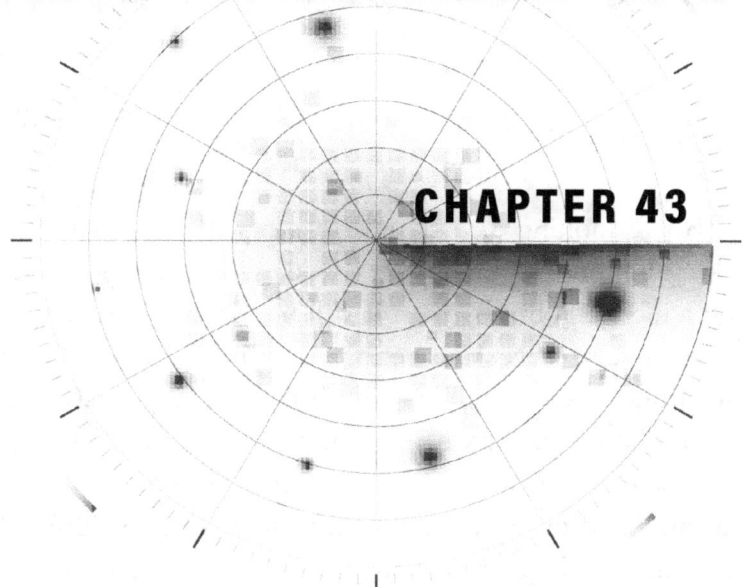

# CHAPTER 43

# VISION QUEST

*Perception is strong and sight weak. In strategy it is important to see distant things as if they were close and to take a distanced view of close things.*

—MIYAMOTO MUSASHI, *THE BOOK OF FIVE RINGS*

his is one of my favorite quotes. Musashi is talking about two types of vision: one type puts your brain in one head space, and the other in another. One allows you to harness your innate, God-given reflexes; the other won't, but it is designed to take in detailed visual information. Both are useful and necessary, but depending on the situation and circumstances, one of the two will be preferable.

This is why, when you're trying to walk with an open cup of coffee or tea without spilling its scalding contents, you have little success if you're looking directly at the cup with focal vision. Everything else is a blur, and you'll miss that dang Lego, or you'll stub your toe on a table leg, but by then it will be too late. The successful waiter, waitress, and server uses peripheral vision to take in as much of their surroundings as possible while also remaining aware of the cup and its level positioning within their peripheral field. This way, they can also take in the steps or the transition from tile to carpet and move around people, pets, chairs, and tables without spilling a drop.

This is perhaps what Musashi was hinting at when he was talking about looking at things from a small scale and a large scale—and everything in between—while also throwing out some deeper philosophical "stuff" this advice on seeing can nudge us toward.

The two types of seeing are focal and peripheral (see Figure 1). Without getting crazy regarding eye anatomy, when we're talking about focal vision, this includes the macula region of the retina, where the fovea centralis (or, simply, the fovea) is located. This central area of the eye is responsible for taking in sharp central vision (for our purposes, just think of this as focal or central vision). It's extremely important to understand the limitations of focal vision and what it does, or forces to happen, in your brain. Focal vision is only about three degrees wide in a beam or tunnel (tunnel vision) directly in front of your eye(s) in the direction you're looking in. We do this when we're trying to read a sign up the interstate, or when we need to see if the street coming up is where we need to exit. We also do this when we're looking at our phones, reading a text, or watching the latest hilarity on Instagram or TikTok. Know that, when you do this, it causes your visual attention to narrowly focus to a field of no greater than three degrees outside of what you're focusing on. This causes inattention and blindness outside of your narrow field of view, whereby someone could approach you—even from the direction you're facing in—and you won't notice them until you look up and break that focal vision to take in your surroundings.

**Figure 1**

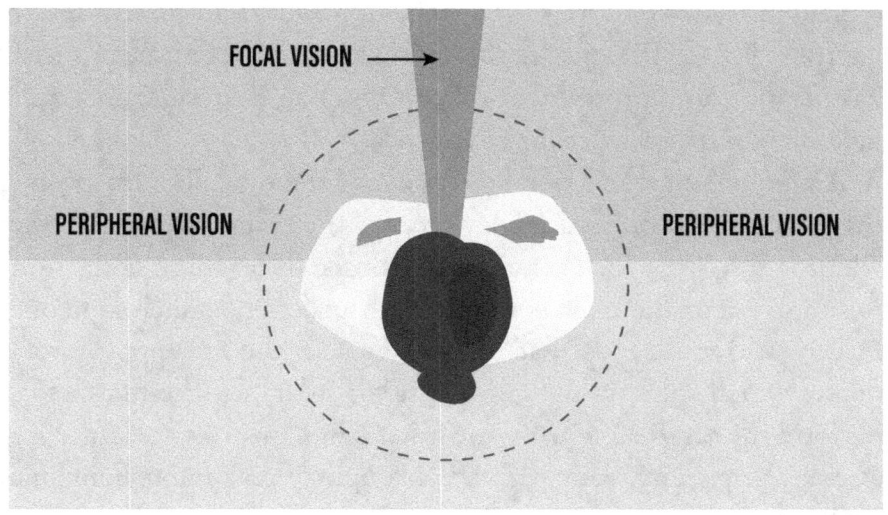

Breaking focal vision opens up your peripheral vision, which is the opposite of focal vision. This type of seeing takes in a wider field of vision, 180 degrees from left to right (if both eyes work optimally), while looking in a forward direction.

Each type of seeing uses one of two parts of the mind: the conscious for focal and the subconscious for peripheral. This is the difference between reading and taking it all in. You must be in a conscious state of mind to take in focal visual information in order for your brain to interpret what it is seeing. Moving your eyes by scanning breaks any potential tunnel vision and opens your awareness back to a peripheral field of view. Peripheral vision lives in the subconscious state of the mind and visually takes in more information but in less detail, focus, and sharpness. This is where we're wired to visually pick up movements, even subtle ones, to then shift our focus to sharp central vision to determine if the movement we caught out of the corner of our eye is, in fact, a damned saber-toothed tiger hiding behind that bush ready to pounce. The reason peripheral vision lives in the subconscious is so that we can harness our reflexes to protect ourselves in a fight-or-flight response. If we remain in a conscious state of mental attention, we cause responsive lag time. This is the old "action versus reaction" conundrum that has plagued law enforcement officers, fighters, martial artists, self-defense experts, and victims of violence.

Action will beat reaction 99 percent of the time. The reason for this is that action only takes a few steps in the brain compared to the additional steps needed for a typical conscious reaction. For action to simply occur, the brain comes up with an action (punch someone in the face) and sends that neural signal to the efferent (motor) nerves which then translate this action (order) for the muscles to perform the act. Reaction, on the other hand, involves at least twice as many steps. Let's stick with the example of reacting to someone who is trying to punch us in the face. As the reactor to the incoming punch, I have to visually detect that the punch is coming, which occurs through my afferent (sensory) nerves, i.e., "Hey, Numb Nuts! This dude is trying to punch us in the freaking face!" This information goes to the brain, and the brain must then formulate and calculate a response. Once an action is decided upon (and we better hope it's quickly decided), the brain then has to add the action for the execution, i.e., send this response directive out to the motor nerves to give the command for the muscles to act (which is all the face-punching dude had to do from the get-go). Thus, reaction has more steps in the process than action, and this is why action almost always beats reaction. The work-around or hack for this is to *not* focus on the punch that's coming at your face, and I mean exactly that: *don't* look at the scarred-knuckle, fist hammer that's whizzing toward your nose. This will force you into a conscious state of mind where there are more steps for you to perceive, formulate a strategy, send the strategy response back out, and hope your nerves fire the muscles to act in enough time. Not gonna happen.

It seems counterintuitive, but you must throw focus out the

window and see as much of your field of vision as you can, which will harness your reflexes. The steps are almost the same for a conscious reaction as for a reflex, but the difference is where you are in your head. For me, the tough part about being a former law enforcement officer and a firearms and defensive tactics instructor was that I was taught to "watch the hands" because the hands (and what might be in them) are what could hurt me. The flaw in this line of thinking is that it forces officers into lag-time scenarios where they are already behind the eight ball and have no choice but to react in the first place. This holds true for most of us in the civilian world, too. Unless we want to go to jail for acting out and punching people whom we perceive as threats before we know their true motivations by allowing their actions to happen, we're all in the same boat.

Reflexes happen without being logjammed in the brain through the conscious mind. Reflexes have all but one of the same steps in the reactive loop as they do in the conscious mind. During perceptions sent to the brain via the sensory nerves, the brain has a response to this information and sends a signal via the motor nerves for the muscles to act. The missing piece is that a reflex has a baked-in response without the need for the brain to come up with a proper tactic, strategy, or action command to send out. Reflexes happen automatically; for example, if you put your hand on a hot stove burner, you'll pull your hand away before you have time to think. Another example is hearing a loud noise or a bang. We usually crouch lower to the ground while simultaneously pulling our shoulders up around our neck and toward our ears to protect this vital and critical part of our anatomy. This allows us to keep bringing life-giving air into our body (by protecting the trachea), protects the means by which we take in food and water (by protecting the esophagus), and protects the huge important arteries (the dual carotids, as an example) that carry oxygen and nutrients to our brain box. All of this is done without thought, just action. The last scenario I'll discuss is a visual stimulus versus the senses of feeling and hearing that were discussed in the previous two examples. You're walking through a field of tall grass, enjoying nature and zoning out a bit, when out of the corner of your eye you catch the movement of a grasshopper headed toward your face. A normal reflexive response is to close your eyes, turn your head away from the movement, and move your hands up to protect your head and face while simultaneously stepping sideways, forward, or backward to get out of the fearsome flight path of this dreaded insect. *Wow!* There are a ton of reactions happening in combination with this set of movements harnessed by your peripheral vision, and they're all done without conscious thought!

The good news is that, through conscious thought, action, training, and repetition you *can* bake in preferred neural response reflexes that don't get bogged down in the conscious "what-should-I-do" trap. Instead, you'll just *do*. It's said that it takes 10,000 hours to achieve mastery. Think of the guitarist who has played for years and years, especially their favorite songs. They can play those songs without thinking, they just *do*, and they manage to stay in tune, time, and tempo. The even better news is that you don't have to wait 10,000 hours or 10 years to get results and to start honing and harnessing this innate human superpower. I've proven time and time again—with multiple participants from martial arts students to corporate employees whom I've taught active-shooter response to—that reaction can beat action by harnessing your reflexes and "looking" at things correctly to enable your reflexes to be harnessed. As far as harnessing your reflexes by using peripheral vision against a potential human aggressor, it is often discussed and practiced in martial arts schools and in certain sports to look at a point along the centerline of your opponent (such as the solar plexus or the hips). This puts the things you're *not* looking at—potential weapons, or their head, arms, elbows, fists, knees, and legs—into your peripheral field of view, whereby you'll have a greater chance of reacting to them reflexively. Enjoy your *vision quest*!

## Exercise:

For the next week, as you go about your daily activities, identify when you're using focal vision and peripheral vision. When you're using focal vision (such as when looking at a computer monitor), move your eyes a bit left and right, let the words or images fade and blur (this often feels like zoning out by looking past or through the screen), and take in as much of your peripheral environment as you can. To shift from peripheral vision to focal vision, visually take in as much as you can peripherally, and then notice or hone in on something in the environment and shift your focal vision to it.

## Bonus:

Notice something or someone peripherally, shift your awareness to them, and then keep tabs on them in this broadened field of view. You could turn your head slightly in that direction from time to time, or look up or down to *reset the peripheral field of view*, but you aren't turning and looking directly at them with focal vision, which means they likely aren't aware that you're aware of them. This can also give the impression that you're under the three-degree focal vision "spell" and looking forward toward your phone, when really you're taking stock of your environment with your badass expanded vision.

---

* Reset the peripheral field of view: The reason you might have to "reset" is because peripheral vision, as stated earlier, takes in more "information" but in less detail, focus, and sharpness. Objects and people can "disappear," but a quick visual bump left, right, up, or down can reset the 180-degree landscape. This visual reset was alluded to in Chapter 34: Ain't No Sunshine, when low-light environments can cause the need for peripheral vision field of view resets to happen more frequently or as needed to keep tabs on what you're trying to focus on.

**Extra Bonus:**

Use peripheral vision when you're doing mundane tasks and not looking directly at what you're doing. I think you'll be surprised to find how successful you can be while *not* being totally dependent upon focal vision. Do this when you're opening the refrigerator to grab a gallon of milk and when you're pouring the milk into a glass. Then put the milk jug back in the refrigerator and close the door using only peripheral vision. Open drawers and doors, grab pens, pour coffee, etc., all while using peripheral vision. You can get very good at this in a short amount of time. For me to take in a quick 360 degrees of my surroundings, all I need to do is turn my head 90 degrees right and 90 degrees left and I can have a great pulse of what is in my immediate environment.

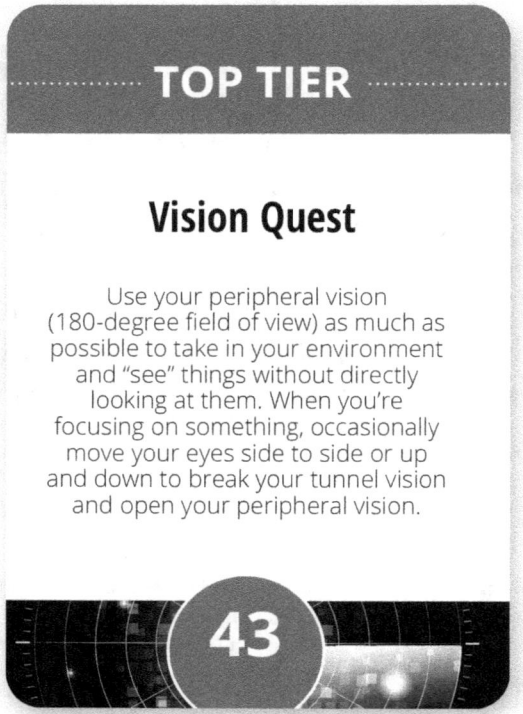

**TOP TIER**

**Vision Quest**

Use your peripheral vision (180-degree field of view) as much as possible to take in your environment and "see" things without directly looking at them. When you're focusing on something, occasionally move your eyes side to side or up and down to break your tunnel vision and open your peripheral vision.

43

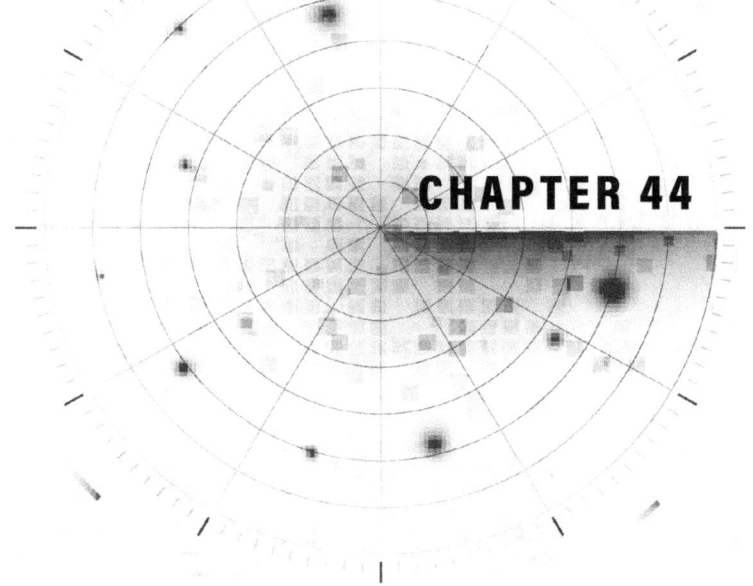

# CHAPTER 44

# LEAPFROG

**B**uilding from the exercise in Chapter 40: Concealment versus Cover, this exercise is designed to form the habit of identifying one or the other and/or both as you walk to and from your daily activities.

### Exercise:

While approaching and egressing from buildings in public spaces, assess what places you could "leapfrog," meaning you could go from place to place. Identify points and paths where you could leapfrog from cover to cover, in order to place as much cover as possible between you and any incoming rounds if you were fleeing an active shooter scene. Don't discount opportunities to leapfrog from concealment to concealment, or any combination of either or both, such as cover to cover, to concealment, and back to cover.

When using a car as cover, remember to think about the vehicle's engine block and tire/wheel axles versus having your feet exposed and hunkering down at the back of most vehicles where the fuel tank is stored. For more details regarding this, revisit Chapter 40: Concealment versus Cover.

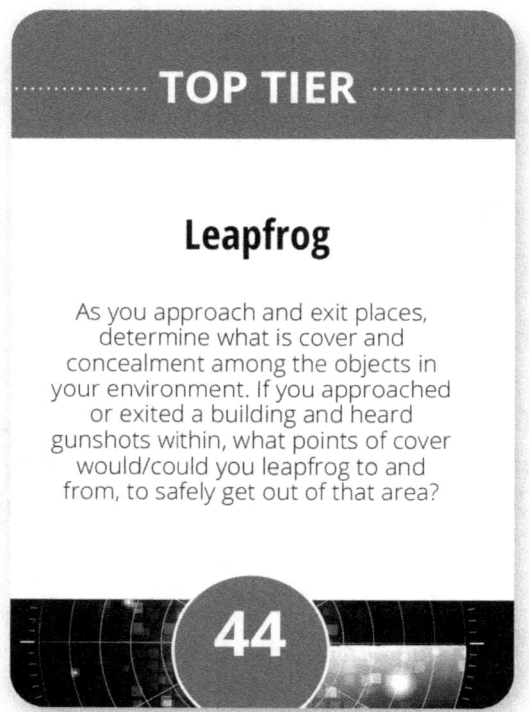

## TOP TIER

## Leapfrog

As you approach and exit places, determine what is cover and concealment among the objects in your environment. If you approached or exited a building and heard gunshots within, what points of cover would/could you leapfrog to and from, to safely get out of that area?

**44**

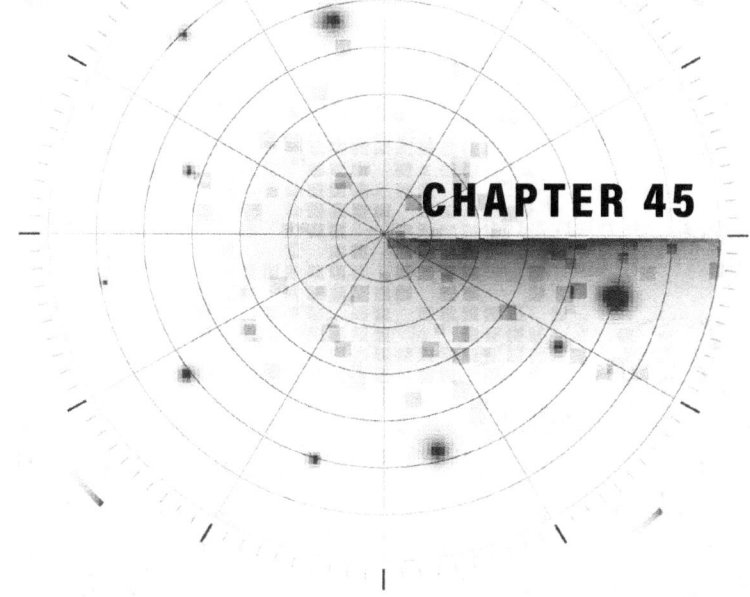

# CHAPTER 45

# OUT FOR CHOW

**D**on't inherit an unsafe condition or environment, if you don't have to. Restaurants are notorious for this. You see the dreaded "Please wait to be seated" sign, and you inevitably get seated somewhere that's not optimal for situational awareness, whereby you could find yourself in the middle of the joint with your back to a lot of action and movement happening behind you. All too often, we don't want to ruffle feathers, seem difficult to deal with, or ask for something, so we just accept what we're given. In a restaurant, the host or hostess seating you offers the table or booth and asks if it's OK. If you don't like it, say so! You're the customer—they should want your business, and they should cater to you. Feel free to point to an empty spot or table you'd prefer to sit at, and politely suggest that you'd rather sit there. More often than not, the accommodation will be made. If it's not, and you are told something like, "Sorry, sir, that section is closed," then you can offer up the next best choice. (See, contingency planning is good!) Or, you can choose to *not* eat there. You have more choices than you think, so *don't* inherit an unsafe condition or environment you're not "cool with."

## Exercise:

Position yourself in a spot where you have the best vantage point to view as much of the room as possible. This way, you can see the comings and goings of folks, as well as the activities of patrons and employees. Don't forget to inventory your exits (from Chapter 1: Exits), which should be gaining "automatic inventory status" in your badass brain by this time (week nine, if you started with chapter 1 during week one).

## Things to Consider:

Later on, in Chapter 48: The What-If Game, you'll want to incorporate this lesson again when you're out at a restaurant. Also, don't forget Chapter 40: Cover versus Concealment. I like sitting at tables that aren't mounted to the floor, so they can be "tumped" over to provide temporary cover/concealment if necessary. "Tumped" is my Texas-ism combination word for "dump" and "tip," as in, "Tump over that table and git behind it!" Please feel free to use it; I'm not going to license, trademark, or copyright it in association with this product line! Tables are my preferred type of seating. I *hate* booths for two reasons: 1) They are almost always mounted to the floor or the wall, so they can't be tumped over! 2) The last thing I want to do is have to "shimmy" sideways like a sand crab across the faux-leather, Naugahyde bench seat to get my feet under me and deal with a SHTF situation. Time would be of the essence, and being in a booth would slow me down, especially if I'm not in the outside position and/or I have people in my party who I need to help. I like having my back literally against the wall, versus having my "back against the wall" negatively speaking, in regard to a poorly chosen position to work from in a SHTF scenario. Furthermore, I like being in a corner where I can see the widest angular signature (breadth/expanse of peripheral vision) of the room or space. Finally, I like to be near the kitchen, server staff entry/exit point(s), and/or an alarmed exit door which is often overlooked yet is easily discernible with signage such as "Emergency exit only, alarm will sound if opened." These doors (by standards set by the Occupational Safety and Health Administration and the National Fire Protection Association's Life Safety Code) are supposed to open out versus in and should be opened with a push bar for easy exiting. *All good* things to consider if you need to Jack-be-nimble the heck out of a bad situation.

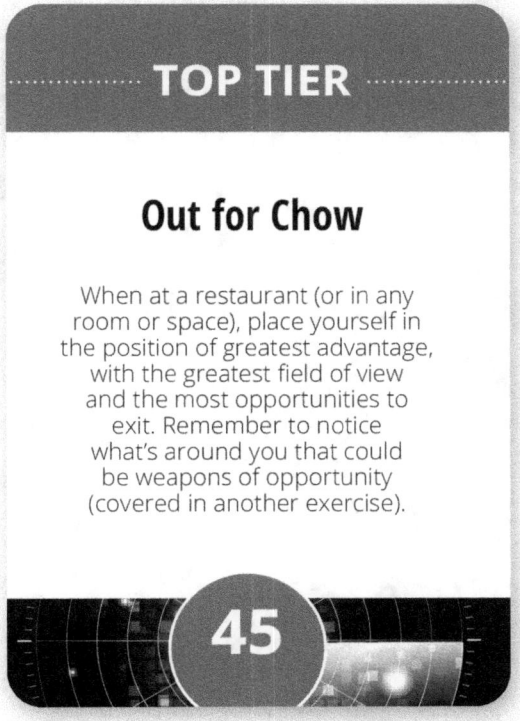

**TOP TIER**

### Out for Chow

When at a restaurant (or in any room or space), place yourself in the position of greatest advantage, with the greatest field of view and the most opportunities to exit. Remember to notice what's around you that could be weapons of opportunity (covered in another exercise).

**45**

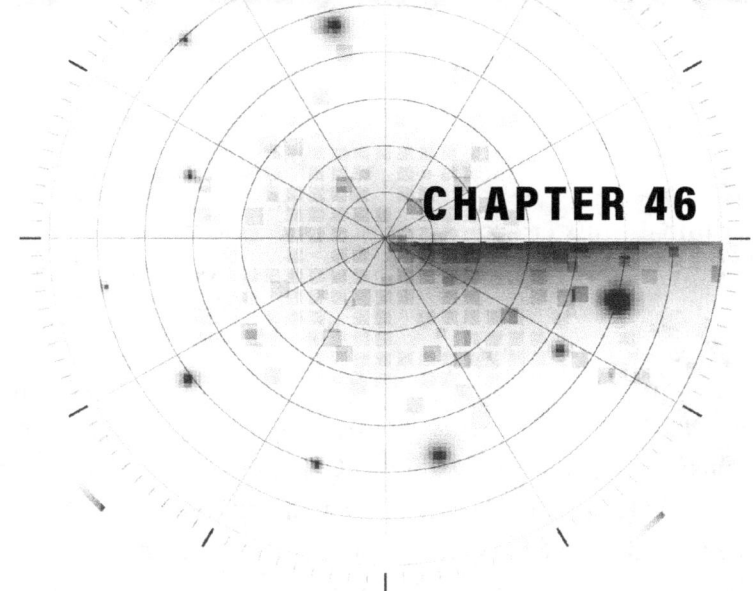

# CHAPTER 46

# WEAPONS INVENTORY

I know I'm not the only one. I make it a point of habit to always have at least one weapon on me when I'm out and about. I do this at home as well, but they're usually not "loaded for bear." For me, it's the ole proverb: "I'd rather have a gun and not need it than need it and not have it." The same holds true for knives, tactical pens, flashlights, etc. I wear these where they can be easily deployed for use *and* I practice in their deployment. It would suck to need the gun, knife, or tactical pen and then have to fumble around trying to get it up and out, ready to defend my life and the lives of others. Practice and reps create a consistent foundation upon which you can reasonably predict or recreate the desired movement when under the high demand of stress. There are a ton of good guys out there who have weapons on their persons for good reasons and intentions. *Know* there are at least the same *ton* of bad guys out there who have weapons on their persons for bad reasons and ill intent. They often will use these to achieve whatever criminal, sinister acts they've planned. Some will brandish them to intimidate and for compliance, while others will use them to do harm.

## ⚙ Exercise:

Weapons on their person: who has them, and who doesn't? This is building upon Chapter 3: Odd Man Out, but now you're looking for fixed knives, OWB (outside waistband) holsters, IWB (inside waistband) holsters, or AIWB (appendix carry, inside waistband) holsters. For those who are unfamiliar with these terms, these weapons are holstered and concealed in the front side between the hip and the centerline of the body, around the area of the appendix if they are right-handed (see Figure 1) or opposite the appendix if they're a lefty. A shirt is usually untucked or worn with an overshirt or a jacket to conceal the holster. Careful observation would reveal its potential location on their person. Look for the common folder knife with an exterior clip exposed outside a pocket's edge. Some people in constitutional carry states (CCS) can carry pistols OWB for all the world to see, and some folks in CCS or with LTC (licensed to carry) or concealed carry permits wear their pistols hidden, usually with IWB or AIWB holsters.

**Figure 1**

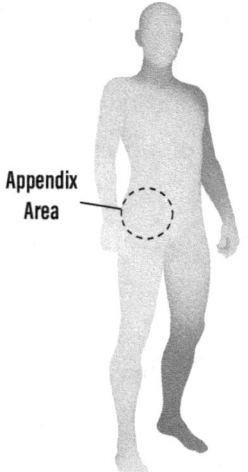

Appendix
Area

When taking inventory, also consider if they have more than one weapon on them. Spot their weapons and where they are located on their person. Do they have things that could be a weapon? That seemingly innocent pen tucked sideways between buttons on their collared polo shirt could be a steel-encased tactical pen that can punch holes in skulls. I often wear these as a backup to a blade I carry, especially in places where you're not allowed to carry a pistol, like at the post office.

## ✚ Bonus:

Can you spot the folks who are carrying a pistol but are trying to hide it? They need to be on your radar! What's your vibe concerning them? Are they a good citizen, a poser, or a creep?

And now, please indulge me in a short rant: There are some OWB folks out there that I have a strong disliking for. Some of these peeps seem to be trying to impress the world with their cheap, nylon OWB holsters with no retention for the gun. Retention holsters have release buttons, snaps, straps, or a combination of these so any knucklehead walking by can't just jerk your gun loose and have it for themselves. This irresponsible safety sin isn't necessarily an automatic deal-breaker for me, as long as they have good situational awareness of their gun side and body positioning, and I may even offer them some slightly begrudging respect if they hover a lower arm/upper forearm across the top of the holster's opening/exit hole. Usually, however, the person who isn't willing to invest in a solid platform to carry their firearm while in public is also the person who did the bare minimum to get a LTC permit and doesn't commit the time and effort to not only train but to train properly with a quality instructor or coach. I often shop at a Walmart near my home in Texas, and I see this far too often: OWB, open-carry pistol dudes with crap holsters that have no retention, and they have no situational or gun-side awareness. These clueless folks often are looking at the shelves with their gun sides facing passing pedestrian traffic while they're reaching for the shelves, making their gun an easy target for a bad person to take and use. Here are a few questions for you to ponder: How many people in America suffer from mental illness? How many people in America suffer from psychosis, schizophrenia, or multiple personality disorders? How many are diagnosed or undiagnosed sociopaths? You can do the math and look it up. I can tell you, it's *a lot* more than *one*—*and* they don't walk around with signs, T-shirts, or ball caps letting the general public know they might have issues. And here are some more questions: How many people in America are on medications, prescribed or self-prescribed? How many people take their medication as directed and on schedule? How many people can have such a bad day that they might do something unexpected that can negatively affect and impact the lives of innocent others? How many people in some of the questions posed earlier could be "off" on any given day? Perhaps they haven't taken their medication properly or as directed. Perhaps they've just experienced a challenging life event that seems monumental and insurmountable. Perhaps they could do something extremely unexpected and violent. Perhaps the freaking knuckleheads with a lack of situational and gun-side awareness, who are toting around an OWB, piece-of-crap, nylon holster without retention on it, could just hand a loose cannon the means by which to create some violence and wreak some havoc! *Rant over!*

## Extra Bonus:

Identify the knucklehead posers with cheap OWB holsters without retention that have poor situational and gun-side awareness—and get the *heck* away from them! Know where they are and keep tabs on them using as many of the tactics and strategies in this book as possible! Bullets can travel quite a distance and can go through lots of things. The last thing I want is an irresponsible, minimally trained gun owner skinning that smoke wagon he's proud to show off to the world and pointing the business end in my direction!

## TOP TIER

## Weapons Inventory

Who has them? What are they? Where are they on the person? Does the person have a weapon but is trying to conceal it? Can you guess if they are right- or left-handed based on where any weapons are positioned? (This might be a wise thing to discern!)

46

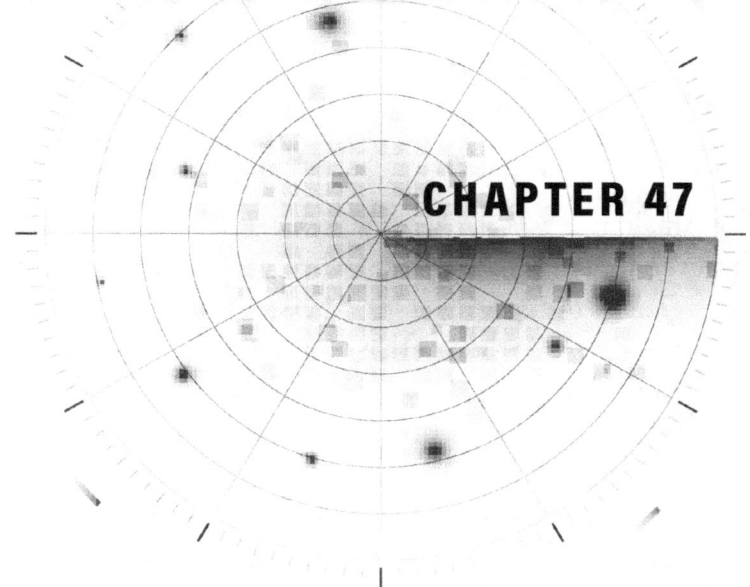

# CHAPTER 47

# MIRROR, MIRROR ON THE WALL

I t's time to reflect.

## ⚙ Exercise:

Scan your mirrors before you exit your vehicle. You can even use the cool joystick, too! Note that mirrors still have blind spots, so Vision Quest it (chapter 43) with peripheral vision as well. Do this every time you exit your vehicle for the next five days. Also know where the blind spots are. But this is just the beginning! Use mirrors, windows, monitor screens, fish aquariums, high-gloss tile on a wall or floor, etc. to take measure of a room and keep tabs on creeps without giving away that you're watching them. The point of using reflective surfaces is that your head is facing one way, giving the appearance that your focus is in that general direction when in actuality it isn't.

An alternative is to wear dark sunglasses whereby you can appear to be looking in one direction when you're actually cutting your eyes as far left or right as possible without moving your head while taking in visual info. I used to work with a buddy who wore transitional prescription sunglasses. He was a master of wearing shades and appearing to look in one direction with his head facing a certain area while his shifty eyes were cutting far left or right to check out hot chicks. The hilarious part was, after he got prescription transitional lenses, we'd go out for lunch together, and he'd forget that his shades had lightened up in the indoor environment and you could see his eyes! It took me three or four reminders and saying, "Hey, creeper, I can see your eyes checking out the ladies...bet they can, too," before he broke himself of this habit, but only when he wore the transitional lenses!

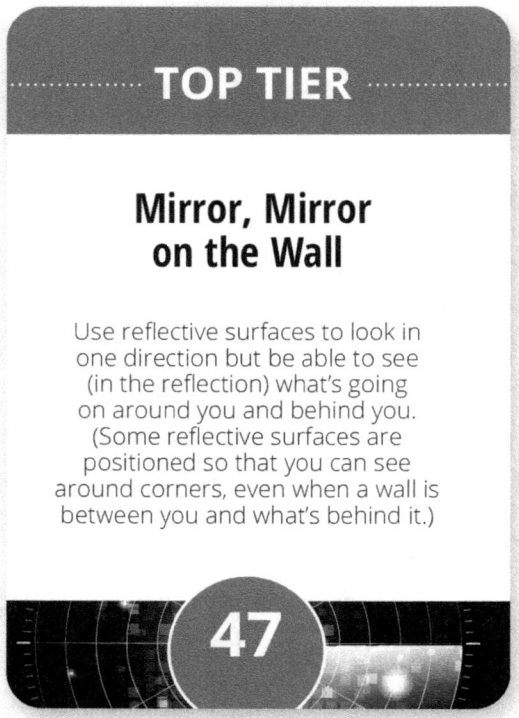

## TOP TIER

### Mirror, Mirror on the Wall

Use reflective surfaces to look in one direction but be able to see (in the reflection) what's going on around you and behind you. (Some reflective surfaces are positioned so that you can see around corners, even when a wall is between you and what's behind it.)

47

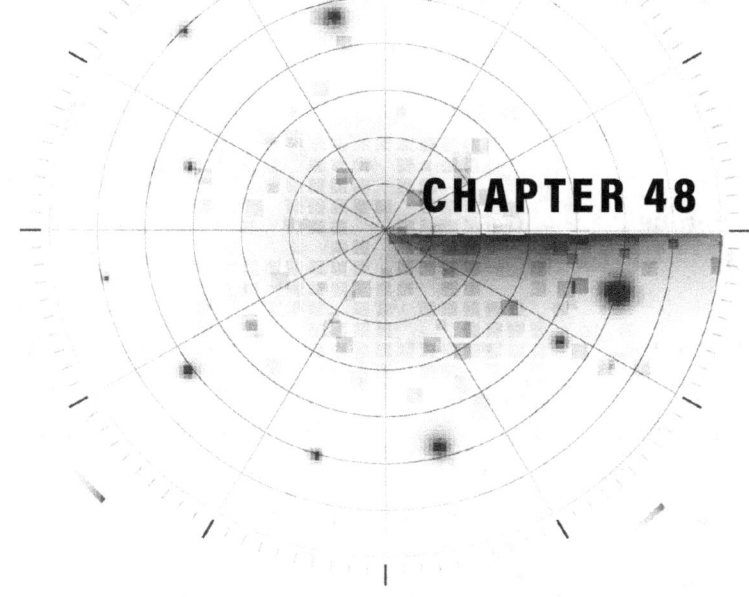

# THE WHAT-IF GAME

(Though it's not a game.) If this happened, where would I go? What would I do? When I'm teaching active shooter courses for companies and civilians, this is visualization at its highest level. It's a mental bullet in the chamber, ready to fire if needed. Plan A, B, and C contingencies. Take inventory—weapons of opportunity—even if you have some good tools on you. It's important to talk here about visualization. True visualization requires vivid imagination if you're going to have any chance of success with it. Visualization coupled with imagination should really put the practitioner in the *experience* of the visualization. This means living in it with all your senses *and* emotions. Make your visualizations as real as possible, include each of the five major senses (sight, sound, feel, smell, and taste), and include feelings and emotions in your visualization. Athletes have done this with success for decades, visualizing themselves running that race, shooting that buzzer-beating three-point shot in a basketball game, scoring the winning goal, and swimming that world record-winning race. The success of these athletes when properly applying visualizations to their workouts and training regimens is evident in top-tier sports icons and Olympic athletes who admit to this being part of their preparation and process for their achievements. Regarding feelings and emotions, always anchor the end of your visualization with a positive emotion, such as the emotion and feeling of success. If visualizations are done properly and you're truly in the experience (as with some of the examples in the suggested exercises to follow), it wouldn't be uncommon to experience a rapid pulse, a rise in adrenal levels, and a heightened sense of awareness when performing and coming out of the visualization.

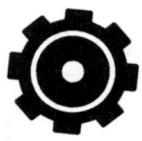 ## Exercise:

During the week, pick places and times to "what if, but then."

**Day 1—At a Restaurant:** A man walks in the front door and starts shooting randomly in all different directions. Where do you go, and what do you do?

**Day 2—At Work:** You're in your office or cubicle, typing away, and you hear gunshots from another side of the building, but you can't see the gunman. Where do you go, and what do you do? If you work from home, get creative. Imagine you hear sirens getting louder and coming toward your street, or you hear a car crashing into some vehicles parked along your street. Or you see two guys jumping out of a car, one flees across the street and the other heads toward your house and jumps the fence into your backyard as police squad cars come screeching to a stop in front of your place. Where do you go, and what do you do? And here's a little nuance to the above, if you're in an apartment, duplex, etc. Imagine the same scenario as above, but the one suspect runs toward your building, floor, etc., and soon afterward, the squad cars pull up and you hear someone on the other side of your door trying to open it. Where do you go, and what do you do?

**Day 3—In Public:** You're in a restroom and you hear a massive explosion not far off that rocks the building, shaking it and shuddering it. The power goes out. Where do you go, and what do you do?

**Day 4—While Driving:** You're passing an eighteen-wheeler semitrailer (or it's passing you) when one of its outside tires blow. The rubber shreds sling off of the rim and slap the front of your windshield. Where do you go, and what do you do?

**Day 5—Road Rage:** Someone is riding your bumper, and as they pass you with all their impatience, they honk, flip you the bird, and pull in front of you. They then start and stop, braking hard in front of you and forcing you to brake to avoid rear-ending them. Where do you go, and what do you do?

## TOP TIER

### The What-If Game

Think of what-if scenarios and mentally walk through how you would react. Visualization with imagination using your five senses is key for success. (If you have family, friends, or loved ones with you, this might change how you would react. Work out these what-ifs, too.)

48

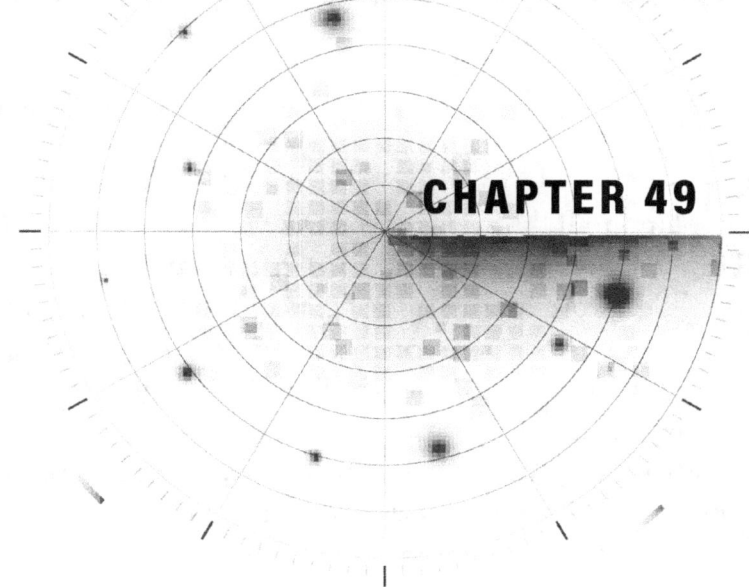

# CHAPTER 49

# WEAPONS OF OPPORTUNITY

They are everywhere!

### Exercise:

In multiple places you find yourself in during each day of the week, scan for any and all weapons of opportunity that could be readily at hand, such as soup cans, broom handles, coffee mugs, pens, etc. Do this even if you're armed! The folks you're with might not be.

### Things to Consider:

What can be thrown? When was the last time you practiced throwing, or actually threw something? (You might be great at it, or you might suck at it! Keep this in mind if it's a go-to scenario or solution.) If throwing is a consideration, I often think about what I can throw, and at what in the room, that might create a big distraction. I'm pretty sure I can wing a coffee mug at that 1,000-gallon fish tank to spiderweb some glass and turn some heads, and if it starts leaking water all over the floor, that might just be what I was "aiming" to do.

What can you grab, and where is the best place to put it "in" a human for maximum effect in a life-threatening situation? Pens are excellent for the eyes, throat, ears, and other soft targets but not so much for the chest and hard, bony areas, or for well-muscled areas on the human body. FYI: tactical pens can be excellent for both soft and hard targets.

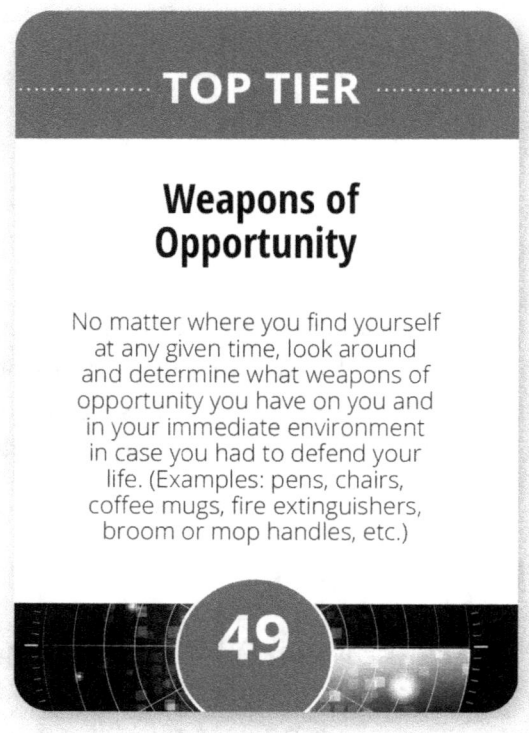

## TOP TIER

### Weapons of Opportunity

No matter where you find yourself at any given time, look around and determine what weapons of opportunity you have on you and in your immediate environment in case you had to defend your life. (Examples: pens, chairs, coffee mugs, fire extinguishers, broom or mop handles, etc.)

49

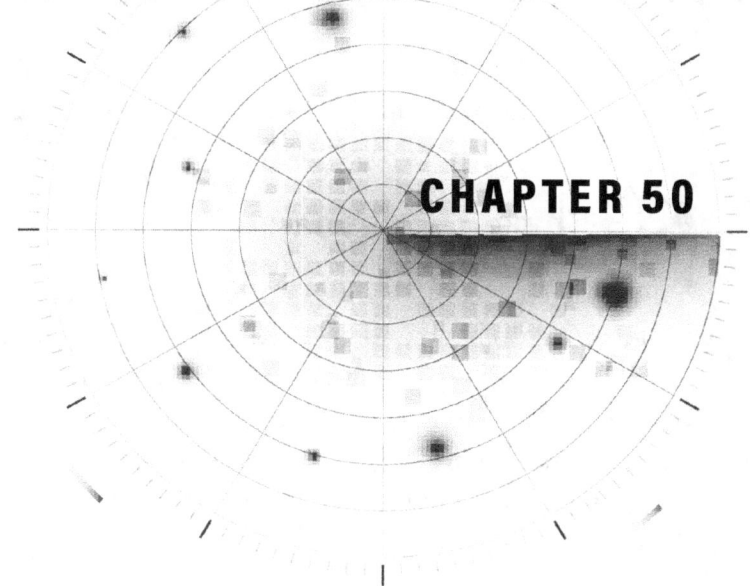

# CHAPTER 50

# A-HOLE HOUR

The a-hole hour extends from 10:30 p.m. to 5:00 a.m. (It's a *long* hour.) Decent people stay inside at decent hours if they have regular work schedules. Heading to the convenience store located next to a bar at closing time to snag that Slurpee probably ain't the brightest idea.

## Exercise:

This week's assignment is to stay at home five nights out of the week during the a-hole hour. If you happen to be out and about during this time, read the following section for some things to consider.

## Things to Consider:

If you happen to be out and about during the a-hole hour, fuel up beforehand and have the provisions you'll need (food, water, etc.) so you won't be inclined to stop after the late movie, concert, etc. This is also a good time to revisit Chapter 15: Case the Joint as you'll be driving by stores, restaurants, and people—but not stopping!—to realize why it's unwise to be out and about during the a-hole hour.

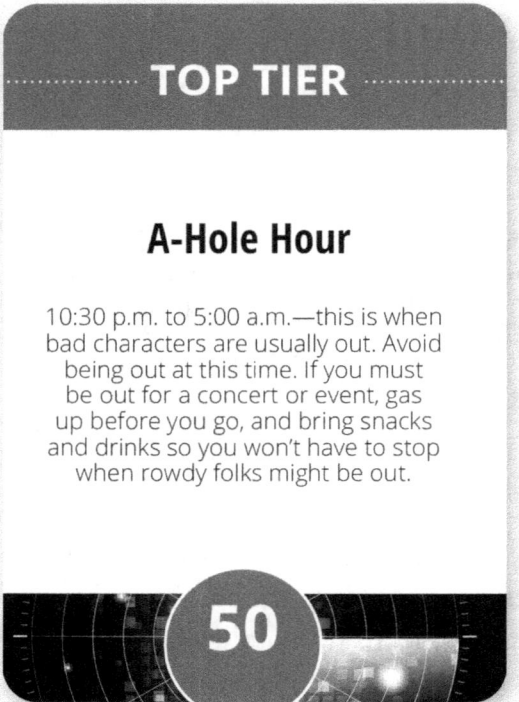

**TOP TIER**

### A-Hole Hour

10:30 p.m. to 5:00 a.m.—this is when bad characters are usually out. Avoid being out at this time. If you must be out for a concert or event, gas up before you go, and bring snacks and drinks so you won't have to stop when rowdy folks might be out.

**50**

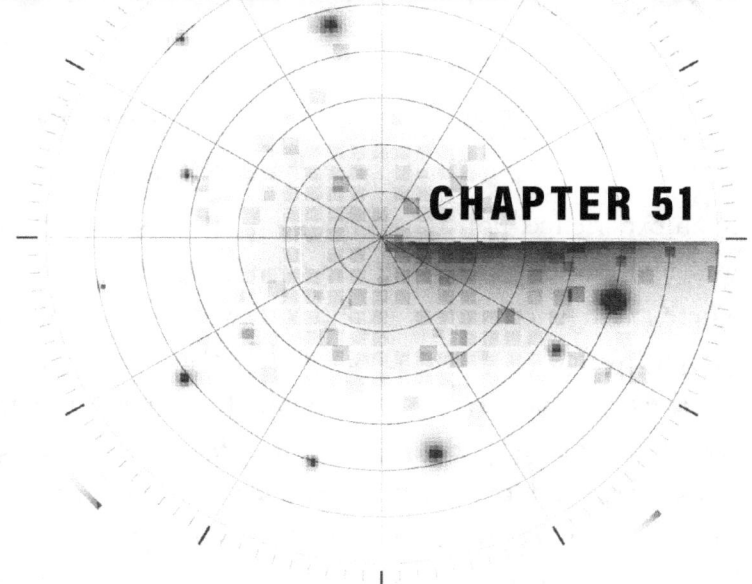

# CHAPTER 51

# REVERSE ENGINEER

**T**hink of the most inconvenient place, space, and time to have to react to a man-made or natural violent event, and reverse engineer it from there. Pick one each day and reverse engineer the tools, tactics, principles, and thoughts to minimize the negative outcome. Use visualization and anchor with positive emotions, even when Murphy (chapter 35) shows up! For me, this would be when I'm going to the bathroom in a public place; taking a shower at the gym, a hotel, or at home; on an airplane; or having sex with my awesome wife.

This is more of a mental exercise than a physical one because the sky is the limit when it comes to your thinking. This can—and should—be done after something has happened and you can think back to any opportunities for improvement that could/should have made the experience more successful. This is often called an after-action report (AAR), postmortem, or any number of phrases that capture the essence of making things better based on the outcome of an experience. For me, obviously, I call this reverse engineering. It is a good idea to go back along the timeline because you can see where the friction points were and learn from them, not only for similar future events and scenarios, but also for potential unexperienced events that have yet to happen. This is where the mental exercise comes into play. Before we hop into the mental aspects of this week's exercise, let's look at an experience or event and use an AAR to improve things for next time. This can be as simple as going to the grocery store or going on a family vacation that had opportunities for improvement to help you survive a scary natural disaster in your area.

As an example, I'll break one of these down in simple terms, without going full-out with the details for some thoughts, lessons learned, and action items for the next time.

- Grocery Store
  - Opportunities:
    - Almost ran out of gas.
    - Low phone charge.
    - The store was super busy, not the best time to shop; caused some unnecessary stress.
    - Key things on the list were overlooked and another follow-up trip will have to happen the next day to get needed essentials.
  - Action Items for Next Time:
    - Make sure there is enough gas in the tank to get to and from the store (unless stopping along the way as part of your errand is part of the plan).
    - Make sure your phone is charged, and have a handwritten note with your grocery list as a backup in case your phone goes down (charged or not).

- Determine days and times of the week when the store is less crowded, and plan your trip around these times so that you can have a less stressful experience.
- Essentials shouldn't be missed based on the second bullet point above; however, these items could be out of stock or otherwise unavailable in the brand, size, portions, or containers you'd prefer. Know what wiggle room you have regarding these essentials and what substitutes could be purchased instead to meet the spirit of the list regarding essentials; this will save you from making that dreaded trip back to the store on the following day. (Hint: toilet paper inventory is always a good idea before you head out the door!)

Once you get good at postmortem and AAR exercises, reverse engineering will allow you to gain the ability to look ahead at what could go wrong and then reverse engineer good solutions and stop-gaps ahead of the problem(s). Chapter 35: Murphy's Law is another exercise to help you execute any exercises from this chapter.

The mental part of this is reverse engineering. Think of the most inconvenient times, places, and/or spaces you could find yourself in when the SHTF and you then have to handle business anyway. Whether it's in public places, in the private sector (such as at work), or when at home, *one* of these places for me would be when I'm dropping a deuce (having a bowel movement, if you aren't familiar with that term). This is a time and place of vulnerability because you'll literally be caught with your pants down, and you'll have to get up and go in order to handle business. Think of all the situations, scenarios, and needs for immediate action that would get you up, off, and running while you're dealing with things "dirty-legged." (Yes, I said "dirty-legged.") There are many situations I can think of that would override the need and desire to take a few swipes of toilet paper across my backside and would require me to handle immediate business dirty-legged. For example, if I were at home, it would be a break-in or a home invasion. If I was in public or at work, it would be hearing the sound of an explosion or gunfire in close proximity; another would be seeing billowing smoke entering the restroom. As I mentioned earlier, this puts a mental bullet in the chamber, ready to fire and act upon when these triggers occur, versus trying to think of the right thing to do in a high-stress environment in real time and creating lag time in the process. Time won't be a luxury you'll have in these scenarios, so you better have your get-up-and-gos mentally baked in beforehand. As a reminder, handling business dirty-legged isn't the end of the world, unless it actually is the end of yours; but in that case, you handled your biz as a hero would and should, and excretion of the bowels and bladder happens in the throes of death anyway, so you were more than likely gonna be found with poopie pants, anyway. Should you come out the other side with a heartbeat and the promise of some more time on this earth, you can always take a shower later, and clothes can be washed.

To be transparent, and to hopefully get your creative thinking in "operator" mode, I'll share two more of my scenarios where it would totally suck to have to handle business. They are:

- Taking a shower or bath (at home, in a hotel, or while visiting family or a friend):
  - Yup, now I gotta run and gun and handle biz in my birthday suit. It worked as a distraction and intimidation tactic with the Celtic woad warriors, and I have Irish blood in my veins, so I'm not too scared of this one. However, one thing I definitely want to consider in my reverse-engineering equation on this front is that I'll have wet feet and will likely be stepping onto a tiled surface. I'll need to be as careful as possible, like I'm walking on a frozen surface, until I can get to that towel, rug, or whatever else I can find to then quickly wipe my feet to get a rough *dry*

to then get my *skin* (the soles of my feet) literally in the game. It would totally suck to hop out of the shower, fully committed to the hard-charging action needed, only to banana-peel slip, crack my head, and knock myself out— or now try to rock and roll with a concussion.

- In the throes of passion:
  - This one would totally suck! But I once worked a case with a home invasion suspect where he admitted to waiting outside windows (usually having cased where the bedroom window was, and on what side of the house) to then listen and wait for the sounds of sweet lovemaking to be in full swing before he and his crew smashed doors and swarmed the bedroom with muzzles pointed at a shocked and surprised naked couple, to then shout commands and start the zip tie and duct tape-fitting process. The sinister nature of criminals knows no bounds, and they will look for any advantage for them during your disadvantage. It's smart for them but bad for victims. I'm not saying you shouldn't *do* what you want to *do* when you want to *do it* or when the mood strikes, but a little bit of forethought and reverse engineering can come in handy so that you're not so disadvantaged. Here are some things I have in place: I live on a decently large piece of property, so if someone is coming over, they know to let us know and to *not* just show up. I have dogs—big ones—four outside and one inside. These are tiers of defense and beasts of nature that have superior hearing, smell, instincts, and other senses that have served and protected them and their packs well and good over centuries of evolution. I am their alpha, and they want to warn me, their pack leader, of any funny business that may be out of the ordinary, should it invade our space. I love them, they love me, and I reward them

when they warn me about something, whether it is bad dudes in my perimeter or coyotes getting too close to my fence line for their comfort. I'm not a loud lover or maker of love noises. Neither is my wife. It's just not our jam; we know how we feel about each other, and we know when and what feedback is good without the need for over-the-top loudness. This was never planned, it just evolved naturally from having our daughter grow up in the house with us at various ages in her life. No matter what you're doing, it's always good to have an ear out. Being in the throes of passion is no exception. Things to further consider in this reverse-engineering scenario is how you set up your bedroom with cover, concealment, obstacles, self-positioning when in performance of the act, and the positional relationship of tools that can be within arm's reach and ready for action if a home invasion were to happen during this inconvenient time. I know some things in this book are rough and tough to consider, and likely there are some readers who will think I'm over-the-top and have too much crazy time on my hands to have thought of so many what-if scenarios, and they might think that's just not the way they want to live. People will live exactly the way they want to live, but how long that would and could be can be very dependent upon *how* one goes about it. Oscar Wilde and Will Rogers have both been attributed with the famous expression: "You never get a second chance to make a first impression." Regarding the home invasion scenario laid out above, and the admission of the captured turd regarding one of his tactics to ensure success, what do you think *could* happen? As a woman, you wake up from unconsciousness, zip-tied and with your mouth duct-taped shut, and your husband or partner is also zip-tied and duct-taped, and you're both naked. Want to speculate on the potential motives at this point? Want to speculate on the motives of the crew and their perverted timing for vthis particular home invasion? Do you think that terry cloth robe is going to be fetched from the bathroom hook to cover your nakedness in a show of some respect for you during this violent act? Do you think they'll sit you beside your partner and head for the jewelry box? Do you have other females in the house? Is there a sleepover happening? Was this random or planned? *Did you think and plan for the what-ifs?* Regarding home invasion scenarios, I agree: "You'll never get a second chance to make a first impression." *I know what I want my first impressions to be!* They will be multiple, on target, and delivered with deadly accuracy.

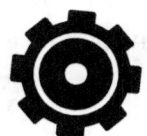 **Exercise:**

**Physical Activity:**

Do an AAR or postmortem on an errand or activity you accomplished prior to this week's exercise but have to execute again this week. Make improvements via a premortem/reverse engineer process, and execute to them. We usually have multiple tasks we repeat on a weekly basis, so it shouldn't be a challenge to come up with and improve upon three to five for this week.

If you're having trouble with action items during this week, I highly suggest you spend some time visiting Fieldcraft Survival and reading/watching anything written, produced, or filmed by their CEO, Mike Glover. Mike and Fieldcraft are dedicated to enhancing preparedness for citizens of all walks of life and in a multitude of situations and scenarios. I'm a huge fan. The time to change those batteries on your flashlights, radios, and other gear isn't when the storm has already hit. You see it coming (so the news is actually beneficial in this context, versus sensational), so go prep—*now*. You don't know how long those batteries have been in those flashlights, so change them now, and get on a battery-changing schedule. Do you only remember you need to change your wipers on your car after it starts raining? Think of all the things you need to do now, and get them up to speed.

### Mental Activity:

Think of scenarios where you would be severely hampered and challenged to have to deal with an extremely unwanted situation. Reverse engineer the snafus and fix them before they can fail, or set yourself up for more likely success, or just go through the mental visual exercise and back in your mental go-to responses so they are readily available should that ever happen. Remember to revisit and use the What-If Game (chapter 48) to anchor in positivity and a win-anyway attitude when Murphy's Law (chapter 35) shows up.

### Things to Consider:

In public restrooms, women have an advantage because a stall is always available, and the great thing about a stall is that it can be closed and locked to give you more security and privacy. For you men out there, my public restroom strategy is to use the handicap stall every chance I can, and I always lock/latch the door. There are several reasons for this:

- When using the urinal, my back is facing the incoming pedestrian traffic. It would take nothing for someone to come up behind me, while my hands are full, and bounce my face off the tile wall I'm facing. I could get stomped, kicked, and (best-case scenario) wake up alive but concussed and missing my cell phone, wallet, keys, and very probably, my gun. It's super easy to walk through a parking lot popping buttons on the fob of a set of stolen car keys to see the vehicle light up and chirp, telling the bad guy exactly which car they can easily steal.

- A stall gives me at least one extra layer to slow down an assault. I "blade" my stance, and I don't stand directly in front of the door because a kicked-in door could act just like a punch, hit, or strike that would wallop me and send me forward. I like to cheat my stance off-center of the end of the toilet (if I'm peeing), away from the hinge side of the door. If I'm bladed on the hinge side, the door could still be kicked open and strike me.

- Another reason why I like to use the handicap stall whenever possible (not trying to piss off anyone here) is because, if I'm going to fight in a phone booth, I want to be in the biggest phone booth I can.

- If I legit have to take a BM, then this is again a bigger place to have to handle business. And since I conceal carry each and every time I can, I like the bigger stalls because the toilet is usually up against at least one side of the bathroom with a wall on one side (not bordered with two stall walls on either side), and the toilet is usually not dead center in the middle of the stall because there needs to be room for a wheelchair. I like this position because of what I do with my gun—if I need to—while I'm pooping. I'm not sure what most people do with their pistols when they're in this scenario, but what I do is an evolution of better decision-making over the years since I started carrying pistols in public at age twenty-two when I was a newly minted Dallas Police Department rookie. What I do now is I sit down, controlling my holstered pistol, and I spread my knees apart so my pants and underwear are tight just below my bent knees. I then unholster my pistol and I lay it inside the hammock or net my underwear has created. I keep the barrel out toward the stall door and canted on the side, whereby my dominant hand could easily grab it if I needed to. The reason I do this is because I don't have a ton of training reps in drawing my pistol from my holster while I'm dropping a deuce, from a sitting position, with my pants down around my ankles. But I do have quite a few reps in drawing my pistol from my appendix position, and this position is slightly nuanced yet familiar, and it's close enough for me to replicate success in a draw, should I need to do it. I also keep my knees spread and the material of my pants, shorts, underwear, etc. taut just below my bent knees so it's a closer and more stable platform to draw from (versus having to fish through some folded clothes, etc.). *And* I don't want to have to draw my gun from the floor, so my pants don't go down to my ankles. *And* I don't want a guy sitting next to me to be able to bend down and spy that I might have a pow-pow nesting in the middle of my tighty-whities that comes with the fashionable yet distinct male, brown racing stripe. (Kudos to my bro Rob who wears black underwear! Smart bro!) Note: If you're going commando (or, for the ladies, if you're wearing a thong and/or it's "that time of the month"), the "hammock," knee-spread approach won't work. Are you comfortable perching that *blaster* on the toilet roll hanger? (Thanks, Mickey Schuch from Carry Trainer! I love that term for a *pistola*!) It would suck for it to clatter to the ground when a person in the stall next to you slams their door too hard. I have actually practiced this with a dry and empty gun. (I know, I know, I have time on my hands...but so do you. How often do you use the bathroom daily?) I have pinched my pistol under my weak-side armpit, between my upper arm and the side of my chest, performed the dirty business, cleaned up, pulled my pants up, buckled my belt, and then relinquished my squeezed pistol hold to then holster my blaster safely back in my kydex appendix blaster holster. The "armpit pinch" isn't all that awkward if you've ever worn, drawn, and practiced using a shoulder holster. If you get cramps, you might wanna hit the gym and do more lats and/or start wearing *black* boxer briefs.

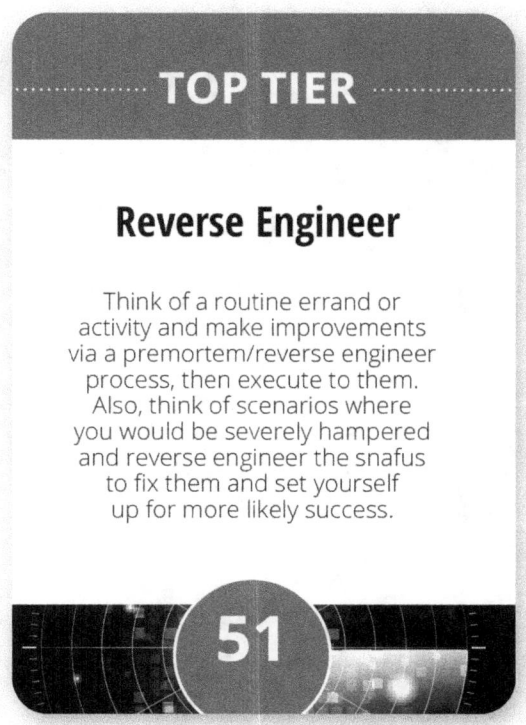

**TOP TIER**

## Reverse Engineer

Think of a routine errand or activity and make improvements via a premortem/reverse engineer process, then execute to them. Also, think of scenarios where you would be severely hampered and reverse engineer the snafus to fix them and set yourself up for more likely success.

51

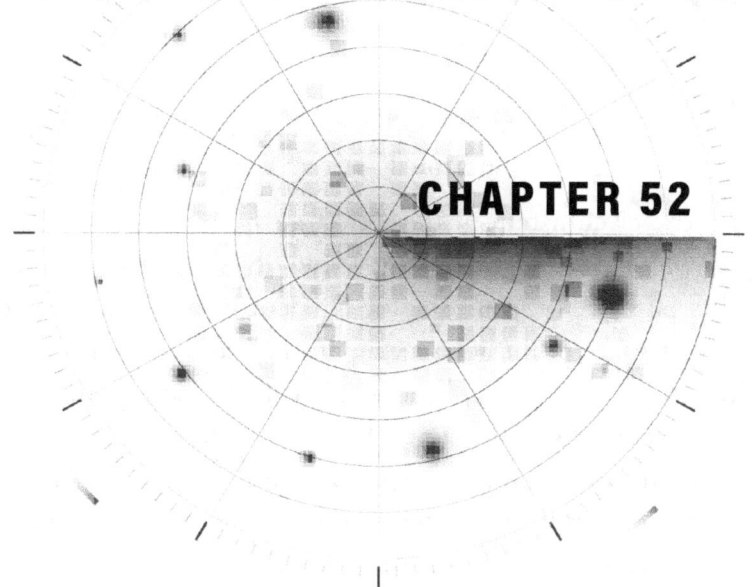

# CHAPTER 52

# ESTABLISH OWNERSHIP

**P**erhaps more importantly, *reestablish* ownership. I had the honor to work for Clint Smith as a firearms instructor at Thunder Ranch in Mountain Home, Texas, and he always said in room-clearing drills, "incoming rounds have the right-of-way." Otherwise, if I "pied off a corner" to a hallway, and there were no bad guys in the stretch of the hallway, and I had to go down this long stretch to get to the next corner, I would have to *establish ownership*. Running and gunning down a long hallway is a point of vulnerability for a team doing a dynamic entry into a building. Clint would say to take it "fast in the straightaways" (hallways) and "slow in the corners," taking sections of the corner slowly, exposing a greater field of view (one slice at a time) to discover what—good or bad—is around the next corner. In operator talk, this is often called "pieing off a corner." This is done to establish ownership of that section or corner (see Figures 1 and 2). If I encountered incoming rounds and had a corner or safe place to step back to, this might be a good idea, depending on the circumstances and whether the bullets heading toward me *might* have the right-of-way. If my objective was to continue down this path, i.e., if I must take this corner to secure my objective, I will at some point have to pie off that corner in another attempt to reestablish ownership. Incoming rounds having the right-of-way is a two-way street. So, when I'm in that hallway and in a vulnerable straightaway, I have to keep the mindset of owning it, and anything coming around the corner(s) at the other end will have to deal with my bullets owning the right-of-way.

**Figure 1**

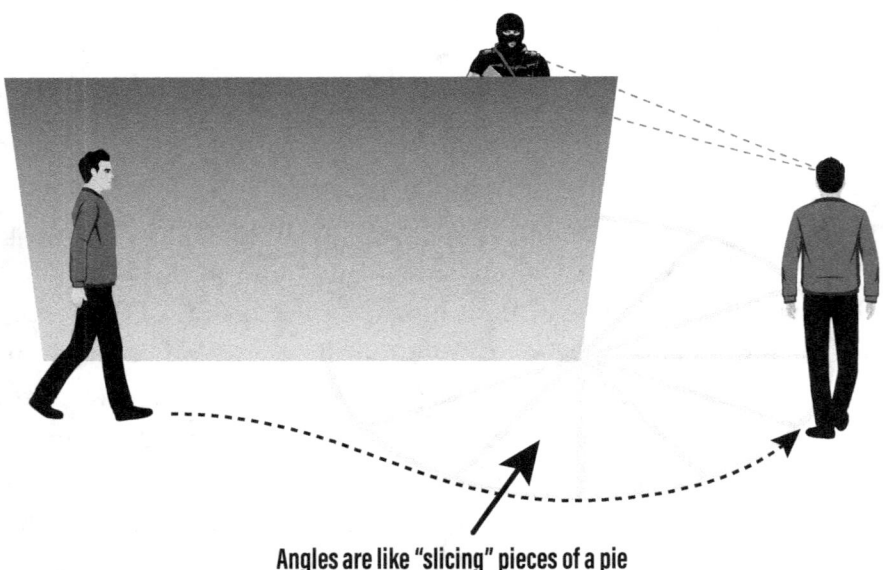

Angles are like "slicing" pieces of a pie

This strategy offers a principle that can be applied to many scenarios in our lives, *not* just building clearing. For example, when driving a vehicle, you would turn your head over your left shoulder to clear your blind spot before changing lanes to the left. The same applies when you've rented a moving truck that has height and width dimensions you're not accustomed to, so you get your butt out of the driver's seat before backing out to establish how far back you can safely go, and so you don't take out that awning in the apartment complex you're helping a friend move out of.

**Figure 2**

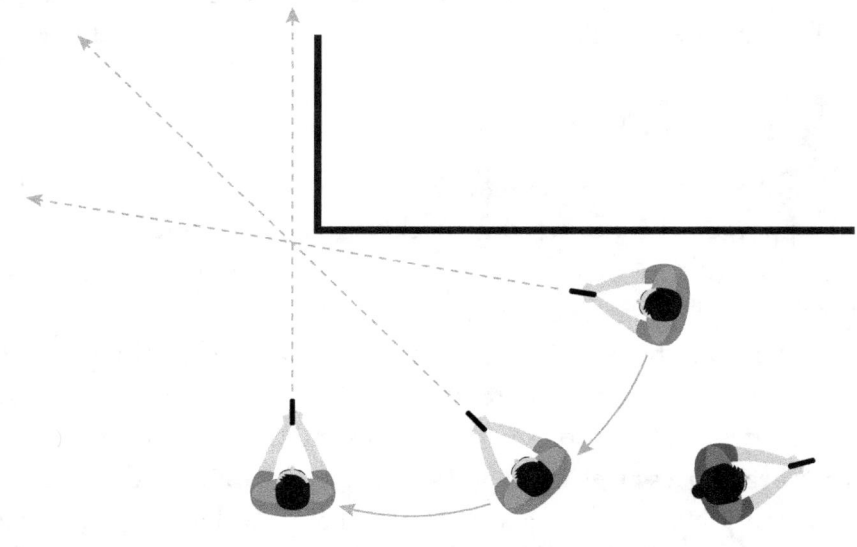

If there is one chapter that I would *top* as *the* most important in this book, then this is the *one*. If you look down at your phone, even for a second, or exit a bathroom to enter a room you were just in, you must reestablish ownership. By ownership, I mean visually speaking. Things can change in a fraction of a second. Even something as quick as looking down at your phone for five seconds to see how many views your Instagram post has, or something more prolonged like having your eyes off of a room while you're using the restroom, can prove a change in environment when you reenter that space. Why? Because time has elapsed, and things could have changed while you had your "eyes off." Are people still where they were? Is anyone missing? Was anyone added? Is that creeper closing the gap and is now ten feet closer to you, perhaps wanting to play Tag, You're It (chapter 41)? Just like room clearing for operators, if we clear a room and leave it unattended, we have to clear it again on our way back through because we don't own it anymore; we didn't establish ownership, which is why, when/if possible, you leave an ace (or aces) in that room to hold and own it, you need to guard your six and give hell to anyone outside the team who wants to own that real estate.

## Exercise:

Establish and reestablish ownership. There will be a slew of opportunities during this week's exercise to practice multiple iterations of this. Before you leave a room, take stock with a mental picture of where everyone and/or everything is. When you reenter, note who might be missing or was added and what things might remain or are no longer there. When driving, you have natural blind spots in your vehicle, so use your mirrors and turn your head (keeping your head on a swivel, like a fighter pilot) to establish and reestablish ownership before you make that lane change or backing maneuver. This is extremely important if/when you've parked your vehicle facing into a parking spot. Things might have been clear when you walked from the rear of your vehicle to the driver's seat, but how many seconds will it take before you throw your car in reverse and start moving backward? In those seconds, the environment behind your vehicle can change quite dramatically. There could be anything from an impatient driver speeding by as they're trying to find the perfect parking spot to kids breaking away from their parents and running past the back of your car because they're excited about the toy run they're about to experience inside the store. None of us wants to live with the guilt of injuring or potentially killing an innocent child while backing a car because we were too *lazy* to check *all* of our mirrors, look in our backup camera, and turn our head *multiple* times to establish and reestablish ownership that we are clear and safe to back out. During this week's exercise, you can also subtly pie off corners, doors, entryways, and exits, and take in pieces of what's around the bend prior to "taking" the hall or the next room, or moving from outside to inside or from inside to outside.

## Things to Consider:

To hone skill on the daily, why not do this in a situation and an environment you might often find yourself in? For example, this may be when backing a vehicle you operate frequently (this, of course, assumes you drive a vehicle on the regular). Thinking about establishing and reestablishing ownership prior to having to do it is smart. Remember the exercise from Chapter 1: Exits, and the lesson on contingencies? This plays into that. To minimize the need to back out when operating a vehicle, think about your exit upon your arrival. Back into a parking spot so that all you have to do when you leave is drive forward. Forward is the optimal direction the vehicle was designed to move in because it has the greatest visibility and much fewer blind spots than when operating in reverse. Backing upon arrival also allows you a shorter window of time regarding a change in the environment. You might only lose two or three seconds throwing that puppy in reverse, validating ownership that it is clear to then back into a spot, versus the five to fifteen seconds of pulling nose-in and then having to back out. Nose-in parking involves you having to open your door, start the car, put on your seat belt, likely plug in your phone, maybe hit play on the playlist or podcast you're currently listening to, and then throw the car in reverse to back out and be on your way. This eats up precious seconds, and your environment can certainly change in that time.

## Bonus:

Pull through parking spots each and every time you can. Some parking spots and lots aren't conducive to this based on traffic flow, angled parking, etc., but some parking lots have two-way traffic in each aisle, and if/when you find yourself with the opportunity to simply pull through two facing empty parking spots to park in the forward position, then do so. You'll easily be able to hop in the driver's seat, quickly establish ownership that all is clear before you put the car in drive, and safely move forward to be on your merry way.

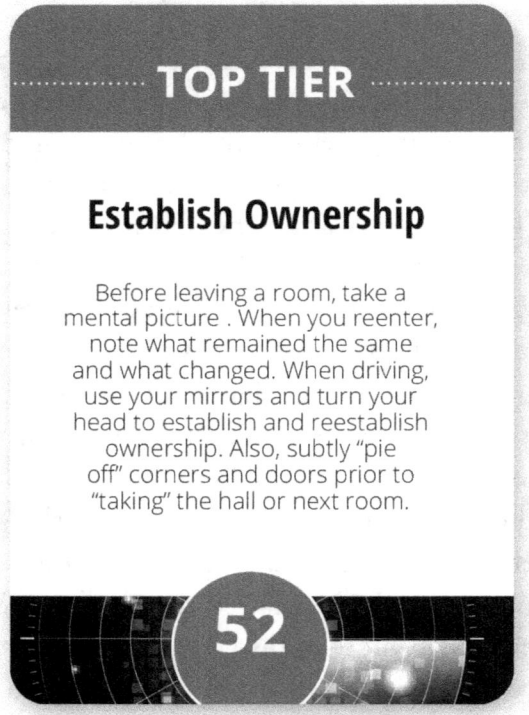

### TOP TIER

### Establish Ownership

Before leaving a room, take a mental picture . When you reenter, note what remained the same and what changed. When driving, use your mirrors and turn your head to establish and reestablish ownership. Also, subtly "pie off" corners and doors prior to "taking" the hall or next room.

52

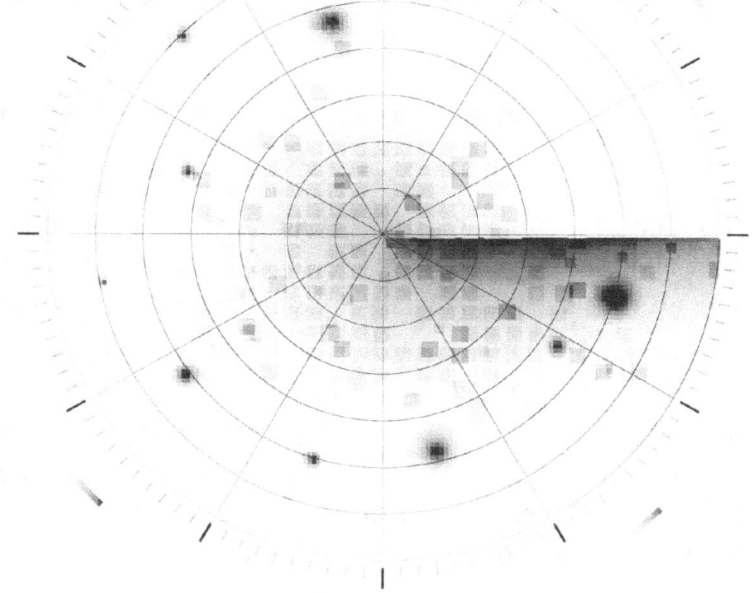

# CONCLUSION

S o, what's next? As I stated in the beginning of this book, regarding the intention of its contents, I hope no one who reads this ever has to use the techniques and strategies in a natural or man-made emergency situation. However, should you have to, it is my absolute hope that this book has helped you better prepare, think, and plan so the best possible outcome can manifest, as opposed to never having been exposed to the actionable tips and drills it contains.

Regarding the levels in the book—basic, intermediate, advanced, and top-tier—don't get wrapped up in any of these exercises being more important than others. They are all important and relevant, it's just that some are easier or less complex to wrap one's head around and execute as drills. I've been taught (and have taught as a martial artist and defensive tactics instructor) that advanced techniques are just a combination of basics that have been strung together in a repeatable chain. I like to think of all these tips, drills, and exercises in much the same way. They can be used solo, coupled with a few here and there, or daisy-chained in a long string of personal awareness exercises that will make you a safer and more secure human who navigates any environment they find themselves in.

Mastery is treading water; it's never a one-and-done. You must keep kicking your arms and legs (putting forth effort and energy) to keep your head above the water line (attain your goals). Skills are perishable, so keep working on, practicing, and revisiting the content to live with more peace and confidence.

One of my goals in creating this work—and I hate that this sounds cliché, but it's absolutely true for me—is the hope that it helps someone, *anyone*, from becoming a victim of violence. When I meet my maker and am potentially told that this book resonated with someone who practiced the material which kept them from being assaulted, raped, and/or becoming a victim of the human sex-trafficking trade, then I will meet my maker with peace, knowing I've accomplished some good in this world.

I want to wholeheartedly thank you—the reader and consumer of this context—for taking the time to read it. I hope that some new knowledge, reminders, and practices have been of value for you. On that note, if you've found it valuable, please share it with anyone and everyone you think could benefit from its contents. Remember: violence doesn't discriminate.

It has been my honor to share some of my knowledge with you. Time is a commodity we all have in limited supply, so I thank you once again for investing yours in this book. It is with my every best wish that I leave you with the hope that this was helpful, insightful, challenging, exhilarating, and empowering to read. Keep treading water!

All my best,

MATT PATRICK KELLY

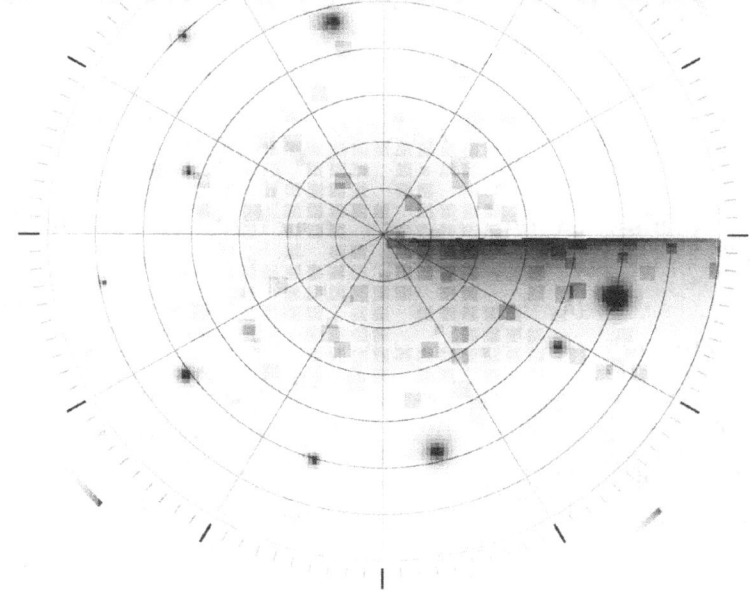

# ABOUT THE AUTHOR

**M**att Patrick Kelly is a Texas native, born and raised. He graduated high school from Bandera, class of 1987. There is not much he doesn't love about Texas and the amazing people in it.

Matt is a former police officer and a defensive tactics and firearms instructor who has also served as a SWAT team member. Matt has been a lifelong martial artist and has over forty years of training and instruction in multiple disciplines ranging from Korean, Japanese, Okinawan, and American arts.

Matt has been a safety, health, and environmental manager for the last sixteen years and has been instrumental in creating, developing, and teaching ergonomic safe-lifting programs, active-shooter programs, and most recently, situational awareness-based training for corporate employees. Matt has a passion for teaching and imparting knowledge. According to him, seeing that "light-bulb" or "aha" moment when someone learns something new and valuable is one of the best feelings a teacher can have.

Matt is the founder of The Knight's Path (https://www.theknightspath.com/), a modern-day knighthood based on the principles of mission, purpose, camaraderie, preparedness, and faith, and whose sole purpose is to provide products and services that benefit humanity. This book is an example of what he feels modern-day knights should put their efforts toward.

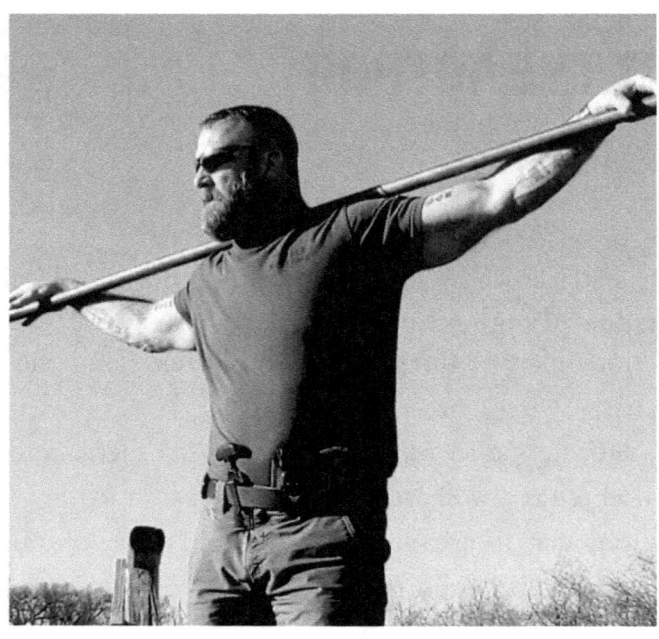

www.ingramcontent.com/pod-product-compliance
Lightning Source LLC
Chambersburg PA
CBHW070656130626
46553CB00005B/1732